The MSing Link

The Essential Guide to Improve Walking, Strength &
Balance for People with Multiple Sclerosis

Praise for The MSing Link

"To live your best life, despite having Multiple Sclerosis, it takes a multi system approach. The most underappreciated disease modifying therapy is exercise. I met Gretchen Hawley during the pandemic after she launched an amazing virtual exercise program for MS. Many of my MS patients have used her program with great success, and I am delighted that she is sharing her powerful information in this text. She is a gem to the MS community and this book will help many families with MS."

— Dr. Aaron Boster, founder of the Boster Center
for MS, MS Neurologist

"Dr. Gretchen Hawley's steadfast commitment and practical strategies serve as beacons of hope, empowering people with MS to embark on their own journey of recovery. Through her many initiatives, she reminds us that exercise and physiotherapy can make a world of difference in the lives of those facing disabilities."

— Mathew Embry, Filmmaker, MS Patient Advocate
& Founder of MS Hope

Praise for The MSing Link

"Dr. Hawley is your go-to MS physical therapist! People at all levels of mobility benefit from her wisdom, enthusiasm, and optimism. This book is full of practical advice for different challenges like spasticity, "drop foot," and urinary problems. Her assertions are backed up by years of experience and scientific studies, and ample pictures show the exercises clearly. Hawley respects the uniqueness of each person with MS and offers solutions for bad days, relapses, and other sticking-points."

— *Dr. Brandon Beaber, MS Neurologist, Author*

"Dr. Gretchen offers a ray of hope to people experiencing MS progression. This science-based book is as approachable and as joyful as Dr. Gretchen herself, and will be an invaluable tool for those looking to increase their strength, balance, and mobility."

— *Ardra Shephard, Writer, Creator/Host of*
AMI-tv's Fashion Dis, TrippingOnAir.com

The MSing Link

The Essential Guide to Improve Walking, Strength & Balance for People with Multiple Sclerosis

Dr. Gretchen Hawley PT, DPT, MSCS

Introduction

When I entered the world of physical therapy for people with multiple sclerosis (MS), my goal was to help them improve their mobility and reduce the effects of symptoms while building meaningful connections with my patients. That was in 2016, three years after working as a physical therapist. This was a life-altering decision. The very first person I treated with MS was a 23-year-old woman determined to build the stamina to stand up during social occasions. Her desire was simple: Go to a bar with friends and order a drink without sitting down. Like many people who face mobility challenges, she isolated herself because she wasn't strong enough to leave her home and walk around with her friends. For the first time, I realized how much most people take for granted. It pained me to see this woman, who was about my age, unable to participate in life in the way she wanted due to MS.

A few of my early patients hoped to walk into a grocery store without looking like they were drunk; or stroll to the pizza shop instead of having it delivered; or escort a bride down the aisle. Quickly, I learned each patient had different symptoms day to day or hour to hour. I was fascinated by this since my favorite part of being a physical therapist is the creativity that's involved. MS requires different exercises and movements for the type of day you're having—high energy, low energy, strong, weak, balanced, and wobbly—and I was excited to work with each patient based on their abilities. However, I didn't feel equipped to do that just yet.

MS is a different beast from orthopedic conditions like back, neck, or shoulder pain or post-surgery pain and weakness. Since the cause of each symptom is different (neurological vs. muscular) it requires a *different* form of physical therapy. So, I dove into the work to become a Multiple Sclerosis Certified Specialist. This was the best way for me to learn everything about MS, and it allowed me to understand the ins and outs of the disease. I was particularly interested in gaining knowledge—and access to—research-based treatments and therapies to reduce symptoms.

In fall 2016, I gave a presentation to a multiple sclerosis support group to educate them on MS-specific physical therapy exercises and techniques. My slides focused on the basics: ways to reduce symptoms like fatigue, weakness, and difficulty walking. I thought, "This is silly, everyone here has MS. They know all of this information. Who am I to educate them on things they already know?"

Frantically, everyone took notes on every slide in my presentation. Astounded is the best way to describe their reaction to my information and the serious gaps in their learning. Simple tips and strategies were not as common sense as I'd thought! And I was appalled that their doctors or other healthcare team members hadn't informed them of these strategies. After this support group experience, I made it my mission to spread as much knowledge and education about managing MS symptoms and utilizing exercises and strategies to notice rapid improvement. If this support group didn't know these simple strategies, it meant the majority of people with MS probably didn't know them either—and that's just wrong.

Many of my physical therapy clients with MS were unable to make it to their physical therapy (PT) sessions consistently due to their fatigue, weakness, pain, poor balance, lack of transportation, and the weather. It gets wet and snowy in the northeastern United States, making traveling to an appointment not only unsafe and stressful, but extra fatiguing. Here's the truth, if you can't (or don't) exercise consistently, you won't reap the benefits. My clients who couldn't make their PT appointments regularly weren't getting any closer to reaching their goals of walking better, reducing falls, improving balance, and getting stronger.

Additionally, most of my clients with MS didn't believe PT could help their symptoms since they'd been down that road before. Or, PT helped up to a certain point, then they'd plateau. Here's why: Traditional/orthopedic exercises don't provide the same life-changing benefits of MS-specific physical therapy. So, I developed The MSing Link, an online wellness program to provide access to MS-specific physical therapy and teach the correct way to exercise. The response to my program was breathtaking. I knew they needed an online resource, but I couldn't have predicted my global reach and impact. MSing Link members (from more than 15 countries) reported, some of them who were diagnosed 20-plus years ago, had never been taught MS-related PT by a healthcare professional. With my program, they improved their walking for the first time in years! They reduced the frequency of falls and climbed stairs with more strength and better balance. Most importantly, they were empowered and hopeful about improving their symptoms, which led to increased consistency with their MSing Link exercise program.

After running my program for more than four years and sharing exercises, symptom management strategies, and research on social media, the next step in my mission was to gather my knowledge into one place. I knew I had to write a book to reveal tools that have helped my clients control their symptoms and improve their walking, strength, balance, and stamina. When all of this is at play, people with MS have a better quality of life.

In this book, you'll learn the essential exercises and strategies making the biggest difference in my clients' lives. I've personally reviewed every exercise, strategy, and tool, which is backed by scientific research. And, I've included lessons from countless MS conferences and discussions with MS neurologists and experts. After implementing The MSing Link's exercises and strategies you'll feel empowered, hopeful, and back in control. One of the most common phrases I hear daily is, "I wish I had this information when I was first diagnosed. My life could look so different!" The sooner you start implementing these exercises and strategies, the sooner you'll be back on your feet (no pun intended) and participating in life again.

Get ready to learn the exercises with proper form and technique. For some, an explanation isn't enough, so I've included photos too. If you'd like a step-by-step breakdown of each exercise, you can find them in the resources page at the back of the book. You'll also learn tips and tactics that'll help you feel more empowered and in control, such as learning the difference between a relapse and a pseudo-relapse and treatment options for each. In the frequently asked questions (FAQ), I answer the most common questions from clients with MS, including how long should I exercise? How do I maintain balance when sitting down or standing up from a low surface? Should I strengthen my stronger side just as much as my weaker side? Be sure to check out the FAQ for the answers, but above all my biggest takeaway is to be consistent and be hopeful!

Let's dive in!

CHAPTER 1

Multiple Sclerosis 101: Diagnosis, Types of MS, and Causes

Multiple sclerosis (MS) is an immune-mediated disease, meaning the body's immune system attacks its own tissues. In MS, the tissue that is being attacked is the myelin sheath, which coats and protects all nerve fibers in the central nervous system. Nerve fibers affected in MS are located in the brain, spinal cord, and/or optic nerve.

When the myelin sheath is damaged (also known as demyelination), electrical impulses from our brain to our muscles are impaired. This causes symptoms like weakness, sensory challenges, pain, problems with balance, compromised cognitive function, and many others. One of the most common first symptoms is optic neuritis, which is when you lose partial or full vision in one eye. However, many of my clients state their first symptom was weakness or tingling in one leg causing difficulty in walking or abnormal fatigue.

MS is nicknamed the snowflake disease because no two people with MS will have the same symptoms. Each individual with MS can have different daily symptoms with varying levels of severity. This means different exercises and symptom management strategies for days when your symptoms are more severe. Some symptoms can be visible, such as walking with a limp, while other symptoms are invisible, such as fatigue and pain.

> The unpredictability of MS causes many people to fear the unknown, but the exercises, tips, and strategies in this book will help you feel more confident in the face of unpredictability.

Let's break down the different types of MS.

TYPES OF MULTIPLE SCLEROSIS

When you're diagnosed with MS, it's most likely associated with one of four types.

1. **Clinically Isolated Syndrome (CIS):** Refers to a first episode of neurologic symptoms caused by inflammation and demyelination in the central nervous system. To meet the definition of CIS, the symptoms must last at least 24 hours. The symptoms can vary per person, but common first symptoms include optic neuritis or any vision change, one-sided leg weakness, or numbness in one leg.

2. **Relapsing-Remitting MS (RRMS):** Approximately 85 to 90 percent of people with MS are diagnosed with RRMS. This type of MS is identified by clearly defined relapses of new or increasing symptoms followed by periods of partial or complete recovery or remission from those symptoms. A relapse is also called a flare or an exacerbation of a symptom. You can think of it as an onset or worsening of any symptom.

3. **Secondary-Progressive MS (SPMS):** If you were diagnosed with RRMS, but have noticed you're no longer experiencing remissions, you may have transitioned into SPMS. This can occur when neurologic function worsens without remissions or when disability accumulates over time. With SPMS, there's a steady decline of new symptoms or relapses.

4. **Primary Progressive MS (PPMS):** This diagnosis is associated with worsening symptoms and neurologic function or disability as soon as symptoms appear, without relapses or remissions. Approximately 15 percent of people are diagnosed with PPMS.

What Causes MS & Who Gets It?

The cause of MS is unknown, however, researchers suspect it's a combination of factors. Possible causes include environmental factors such as low vitamin D levels, smoking, and high body mass index during adolescence. Additionally, genetics, and being infected with the Epstein-Barr Virus (a.k.a. mononucleosis or the kissing disease) are also associated with this chronic condition.

People between the ages of 20 to 50, with an average age of 30, are typically diagnosed with MS. Women are two to three times more likely than men to be diagnosed. Researchers once believed White people were more likely to develop MS compared to Black people, however, a study (2022) led by Dr. Annette Langer-Gould from Los Angeles Medical Center indicated that more Black people have MS than previously thought. The rate of diagnosis is consistent in Black and White Americans. Scientists don't know the reasons for these differences yet, which is likely due to Black people being underrepresented in research, making it harder to find answers. Blacks often experience greater MS-associated disabilities than Caucasians. To participate in research, consider checking out various clinical trials at www.clinicaltrials.gov.

How is MS Diagnosed?

When someone asks, when were you diagnosed with MS, do you say the year of your diagnosis? Or the year of your first symptom? More likely than not, these are very different years. On average, there's about a 10 to 15-year difference between when my clients noticed their first symptom (whether they knew it was MS or not at the time) and when they were diagnosed. Fortunately, the gap is closing with advancements in testing, meaning people are discovering their diagnosis earlier than ever before.

Since there are no specific tests to diagnose MS, a diagnosis is often based on a thorough medical history and examination, various tests, and ruling out other conditions or infections that produce similar symptoms. The examination is performed by a neurologist and includes testing strength, balance, coordination, reflexes, and vision.

Other Possible Tests Include:

- **MRI:** This shows lesions, also known as scars, in your brain, spinal cord, or optic nerve. In order to be diagnosed with MS, your MRI must show at least two different lesions occurring at two different times (greater than 30 days apart). This is the most common test used to diagnose multiple sclerosis when combined with a medical history and examination.

- **Blood tests:** Check for specific biomarkers associated with MS.

- **Spinal tap:** A spinal tap, also known as a lumbar puncture, allows for the examination of the fluid inside your spinal cord, called cerebrospinal fluid (CSF). This fluid shows abnormalities in antibodies associated with MS.

- **Evoked potential tests:** These record the electrical signals produced by your nervous system in response to stimuli, such as electrical stimulation or a visual stimulus. Electrodes measure how quickly information travels down nerve pathways. The slower the signal, the more likely there's a possibility of MS.

You're Diagnosed With MS—Now What?

There are several treatment and symptom management options for multiple sclerosis. If you choose to follow the route of Western medicine, currently, there are more than 20 disease-modifying therapies (DMT) that aim to slow the progression of MS and reduce the annual relapse rate. Other treatment approaches focus on treating symptoms, which can include various diets, acupuncture, massage, electrical stimulation, chiropractic work, vibration therapy, supplements, and vitamins. Other interventions such as hematopoietic stem cell therapy (HSCT) are undergoing clinical trials as a possible treatment. Sometimes, people choose to follow one or more of these options, while others participate in a combination of medication and holistic approaches.

It's also important to see a specialist to address your symptoms. For example, for leg weakness, difficulty walking, or poor balance, a physical therapist will guide you through exercises to improve these symptoms. If you're struggling with hand weakness and difficulty using your hands for day-to-day activities, an occupational therapist may be your best bet. For speech or swallowing symptoms, a speech and language pathologist is a great resource. Discuss symptoms with your neurologist and request referrals to specialists who can treat your conditions. Getting baseline measurements as soon as you're diagnosed allows you to compare measurements down the road.

MS-specific therapies are very different from traditional orthopedic physical therapies since the former focuses on strengthening muscles through neuroplasticity, whereas the latter typically does not. In your search for a therapist, it's best to work with someone who is an MS Certified Specialist (MSCS) or a neuro-certified specialist (NCS).

In this book, you'll learn MS-specific exercises and strategies to improve symptoms such as weakness, poor balance, and difficulty walking, but we'll also focus on improving your confidence and helping you take back control.

One of my MSing Link members, Amy, has experienced physical therapy from a non-MS-specialized therapist and with an MS specialist (me!). She had a great physical therapist, but at some point she plateaued and couldn't push through to the next level of improvement. MS caused fluctuations in her walking, but after being a MSing Link member for several months, she noticed improvements and pushed past her plateau—her quality and speed became more consistent, her endurance increased, and she was able to jog a few minutes on the beach one day! And day-to-day activities and household chores became easier. Her fluctuations in mobility stabilized once she focused on MS-specific exercises, the same ones you'll learn in this book!

Shortly after noticing these improvements, Amy ran into some challenges: illness, anemia, and some unexplained setbacks. This drastically reduced her walking endurance again and decreased her energy and stamina, causing Amy to cut back on her at-home exercises. However, she stayed as consistent as she could with her MSing Link exercises. Later, when Amy's physical therapist measured her functional tests, she was surprised to discover that she had either maintained or improved across all measures. Amy made gains despite a setback. Focusing on this type of therapy allowed her to feel stronger, more confident, and excited for the future. That's the power of MS-specific exercises.

KEY TAKEAWAYS

1. MS is an immune-mediated disease where the body attacks the immune system, specifically the myelin, which covers the nerves in our brain, spinal cord, and optic nerves. This can cause lesions (scars) in those areas, which can result in symptoms with strength, balance, memory, tightness, speech, and more.

2. Women are two to three times more likely to be diagnosed with MS; the average age of diagnosis is in people between 20 to 50 years old.

3. Common treatments include disease-modifying therapies, holistic approaches, or both.

4. Have hope! There's so much research regarding treatments, ways to reduce symptoms and halt MS in its tracks. We'll review these in this book!

RESOURCES

- The MSing Link Podcast Episode No. 84, "Progress Through Resilience w/ Amy M."

CHAPTER 2

Manage Your Symptoms With These Surprising Strategies

MS is called the "snowflake disease" since no two people have the same symptoms. Similarly, each individual can have varying symptoms from day to day or sometimes even hour to hour. Fortunately, MS-specific physical therapy can address more symptoms than you may think. Of course, it can have a positive impact on weakness, balance, walking, and flexibility, which we'll talk about in the remaining chapters, but it can also improve fatigue, sensory symptoms, heat and cold intolerance, spasticity, cognition, and bowel and bladder functions.

Every symptom can either have a primary or secondary cause. A primary symptom is due to inflammation and demyelination associated with multiple sclerosis. Treatment for primary symptoms often includes medication prescribed by your neurologist. A secondary symptom is due to a trigger such as lack of sleep, over-exercising, stress, an infection, heat or cold intolerance, or packing too much into your day. The good news is that secondary symptoms are controllable and managed through simple tricks of the (physical therapy) trade.

Fatigue

Fatigue is the most common symptom of multiple sclerosis, estimated to occur in about 75 to 95 percent of people with MS. Let's call out the elephant in the room: MS fatigue is not the same thing as non-MS related fatigue. Your loved ones may think they know what your fatigue feels like, but they don't. Primary fatigue often feels like heaviness. My MSing Link members describe it as if each leg has an additional 50-pound weight attached to it or their eyelids are too heavy to open. The treatment for primary fatigue is often medication and/or light exercise.

Secondary fatigue feels like you overdid it, even if you've barely moved all day. Secondary fatigue is often treated with light to moderate exercise, energy conservation techniques, organization and planning strategies. I know this sounds counterintuitive. How can you exercise if you're already fatigued? Numerous studies, including research from Professor Farzin Halabchi of Tehran University (in 2017) and others show that low to moderate intensity levels of exercise can reduce primary and secondary fatigue. Any type of low-intensity exercise or movement counts. If you can't get out of bed or you're glued to the couch, perform light upper body movements like forward punches, arm swings, or upper body jumping jacks. Similarly, if you can move your legs, try light marching, leg kicks, or standing up and sitting down. Start with as many repetitions as you can manage while taking lots of rest breaks. Some movement is more helpful than no movement at all.

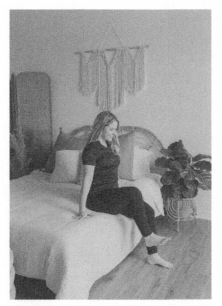

Marching - Bring one knee up toward the ceiling.

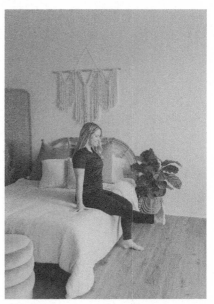

Leg Kicks - Straighten one knee

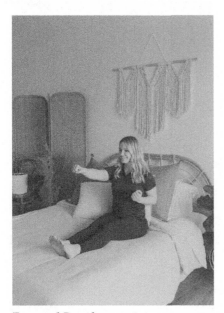

Forward Punches pt. 1

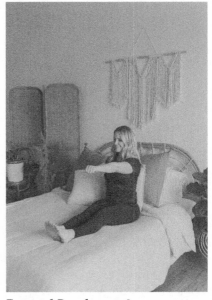

Forward Punches pt. 2

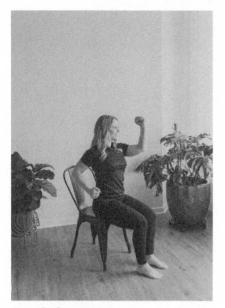

Arm Swing pt. 1

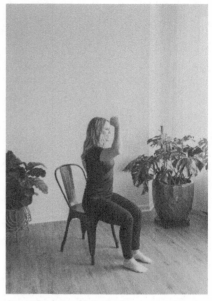

Arm Swing pt. 2

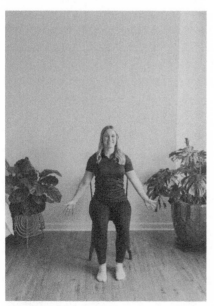

Jumping Jacks pt. 1

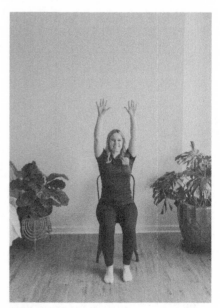

Jumping Jacks pt. 2

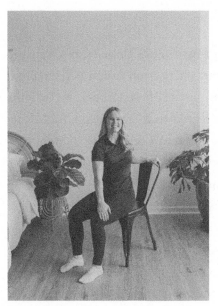

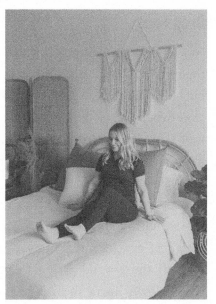

Torso Twist - Repeat on both sides

Heel Slides - Slide one heel toward your bottom.

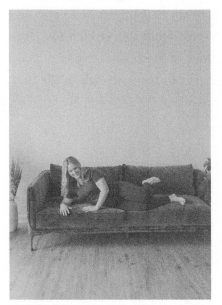

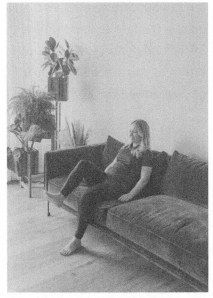

Hamstring Curl on Couch - Bend your knee (you can bend one or both knees); alternate sides

Marching on Couch - Recline and bring one knee up toward the ceiling; alternate on both legs

Drop Foot

MS tends to attack certain muscle groups more than others, causing them to be weak. I dive into this in our chapter on functional exercise, but let's discuss the most common area of weakness my clients experience: drop foot. This is also referred to as foot drop, foot drag, foot slap, or foot/toe scuffing. This symptom occurs due to weakness in the front of your ankle and/or tightness on the back of your lower leg, causing your foot to drop, scuff, or slap. The best exercise to strengthen the front of your ankle is ankle dorsiflexion where you're sitting with your feet on the ground and your knees straightened so your feet are several feet away from you. From here, slowly lift your toes off the ground as high as you can while your heels stay down. Then, slowly lower them. Repeat as many times as you can with good quality, up to 30 repetitions. Make sure your foot isn't rolling inward or outward. Another great exercise to reduce foot drop is a calf stretch. To stretch your calf muscles, stay seated and straighten one knee as far as you can. Use a cane or a yoga strap to loop around your toes on the straight leg and pull it toward you. Hold this stretch for 20 to 30 seconds and repeat two to four times on each side. If you prefer a different calf stretch, go for it! The goal is to feel a stretch in the back of your lower leg.

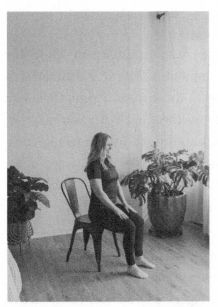

Ankle Dorsiflexion/Toe Lifts pt. 1

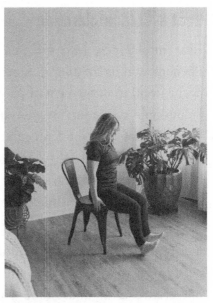

Ankle Dorsiflexion/Toe Lifts pt. 2

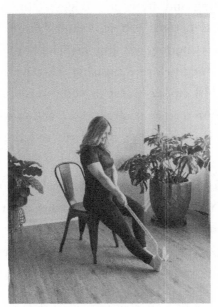

Calf Stretch Using a Walking Stick

Heat & Cold Intolerance

Heat intolerance, also referred to as heat sensitivity or Uhthoff's Phenomenon, is another common symptom of MS. It is estimated to occur in 60 to 80 percent of people with the disease. This is when one or multiple symptoms worsen due to overheating. What you may not know is that heat intolerance is not only caused by the temperature outdoors but it's caused by anything that increases your core temperature by at least half of a degree—that's it! Common triggers include stress, exercise, walking or running long distances, or infection.

Barometric pressure often affects your core temperature. This means you may sit in air conditioning indoors, but it's hot and humid outside so your symptoms still worsen. The best strategy for heat intolerance is to understand your triggers so you can be proactive about managing them. My favorite strategy is to take small sips of ice water before, during and after each trigger. For example, if exercise causes worsened symptoms, sip ice water before, during, and after exercise. Or, wear a cooling vest (my favorite brand is Thermapparel) or cooling wristbands before exercising. However, if you're unaware of your triggers, just sip ice water as soon as any symptom worsens. Additionally, if your trigger is stress, take action to calm your mind. My favorite technique that helps my clients reduce stress is to color in a coloring book.

The lesser-known symptom related to Uhthoff's Phenomenon is cold intolerance. Your symptoms worsen when your core temperature drops by at least half of a degree. When this occurs, take measures to increase your core temperature, by sipping hot water, bundling up in blankets, or moving your body.

Sensory Changes

Sensory symptoms, like numbness, tingling, burning, pins and needles, itchiness, pain, or "bugs crawling" occur in 20 to 50 percent of people with MS. This is most impactful when it occurs in the hands or feet since it can affect your ability to grasp objects without dropping them or feeling the ground when walking. Sensory symptoms caused from MS can only improve with medication or sensory exercises, which is why you won't see any sensation improvement from doing strengthening exercises. The best strategy to minimize unwanted sensations is to desensitize the area by touching it with various objects that have different sensations such as hot and cold, sharp and dull, and soft and rough.

One of my favorite exercises is to roll your hands or feet in a bowl or Ziploc bag of dried rice. This way, you're introducing rice's sharp edges and dull sides. Do this activity for about five minutes or until the sensory symptom starts to lessen. Perform this activity a few times a day until the sensation isn't as present in your daily life. At that time, drop down to once per day, eventually decreasing to once per week. Other possible objects you can use, in addition to or in place of rice are a cotton ball, a soft sweater, a hairbrush, rough fabric such as jeans, a pen cap, or stones.

One of my clients, Katie, had intense burning and numbness in her lower legs. It was too painful to walk. Our regular physical therapy exercises weren't helping on those days, so I poured a bunch of rice into a bucket. She put both feet in the bucket and moved her ankles and toes around in the rice. After 10 minutes, Katie noticed the burning lessened and her legs felt more comfortable. She walked out of the PT session with less pain and she was able to feel more connection with the ground. In order to make a lasting change, you'd need to perform this desensitization exercise multiple times per week, if not daily for several weeks or months.

> Feeling the ground is extremely important when working towards improving your walking. If you cannot feel the ground, you do not know where your foot is when it strikes the ground, which can lead to imbalance issues.

In addition to the exercise listed above, some helpful tools that can help improve sensation in your feet are a vibration plate or insoles designed to increase foot sensation, such as Naboso Neuro Insoles. Information to purchase these items is in the back of the book in the resources section.

Spasticity

One of the most common symptoms that can restrict or prevent movement is spasticity. Spasticity is an abnormal increase in muscle tightness that often interferes with movement and/or speech, depending on which muscles are spastic. If your legs are spastic, walking may be more challenging since one leg might not want to bend (this means your quadriceps muscles are spastic). If you have spasticity in your throat muscles, it can make swallowing or speaking challenging. If you have spasticity in your torso, also called MS Hug, you may feel pain in your abdomen or difficulty taking a deep breath. Spasticity is different from a muscle spasm since spasms release shortly after the tightness begins whereas spasticity does not. Spasticity feels like your limb is heavy and dragging you down. Typically, no matter how hard you try to break the spasticity by moving the affected muscle, it won't move much. Resting the muscle is the best strategy to allow the spasticity to reduce on its own.

Appropriate treatment for spasticity depends on the severity of the symptom. In chapter 7, we'll review the various grades of spasticity which play a role in management of this symptom. Common strategies for lower-level spasticity are stretching, massaging, or rolling the affected muscles. For example, if your knee is "stuck" in a bent position, that is an indicator that your hamstrings are spastic. The solution could be to perform a hamstring stretch; or have someone massage your hamstrings; or roll out your hamstrings on a foam roller or with a muscle roller stick. If your knee is stuck in a straight position, making it challenging to bend your knee, that's an indicator that your quadriceps muscles are spastic. You could perform a quad stretch, massage your quads, or roll them out. When it comes to MS hug, you could try stretching out your torso by performing some classic yoga poses in a chair like a cat/cow or torso twists. Some of my clients are able to reduce their MS Hug from movement, such as punching their arms forward while allowing their bodies to twist from side to side. We'll talk more about stretching to reduce spasticity in chapter 4.

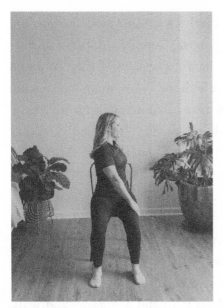

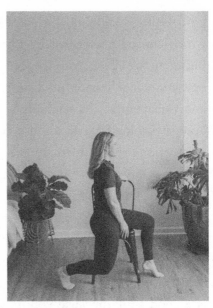

Torso Twist   **Quad Stretch**

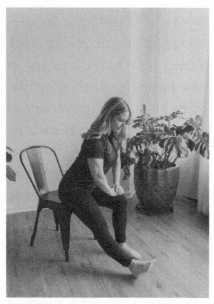

Hamstring Stretch

Other treatment options for spasticity include oral medication, which can be prescribed by a neurologist. Common options include Baclofen, which targets the central nervous system. Other common options include Tizanidine, Dantrolene Sodium, Diazepam, Clonazepam, and Gabapentin. Occasionally supplements like magnesium may help. Your neurologist will discuss which option is best based on other medications in your treatment plan. If oral medications don't help, another option may be botulinum toxin, better known as botox injections. One benefit to botox is that the medication is placed in the exact muscle that is spastic, whereas oral medications are systemic and travel throughout the entire body. Botox injections in the legs are more likely to make you feel like you have "jelly legs." When the stiffness lessens, your true muscle strength is revealed. Sometimes, spasticity is a good thing because you depend on it to stand upright and walk when your muscles are weak. So, if we lessen the spasticity, and we don't have strength, we may feel unsteady and weak. Work with a neurologist to determine which option is best for you.

One of my clients, Pam, had spasticity in her hamstrings that she felt had increased due to temperature changes and stress, so we spent a 30-minute PT session stretching and massaging them. She left the session feeling much looser, but shortly after, she felt wobbly when walking. We used this information during future sessions. We'd work on loosening the spastic muscles slightly, but not fully, so she could use some of the spasticity to maintain balance.

Cognition

Cognitive changes can be common in MS resulting in difficulty with word finding, slower processing speed, poor memory, and attention. For most cognitive changes, it's recommended to work with a behavioral neurologist, occupational therapist, or speech and language pathologist. One cognitive symptom physical therapy can address is difficulty doing two things at once, for example walking and talking. Walking often requires so much thinking for each individual step that it can be challenging to have a conversation or listen to someone talking at the same time. An exercise you can use to reduce this symptom is to practice doing a physical and mental task at the same time. For example, practice ankle dorsiflexion (which you learned above) while counting down from 100 by 3s. Or, practice seated leg kicks while naming everything you can think of that starts with the letter S. This works your cognition and physical body to improve multitasking.

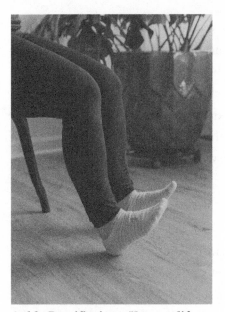

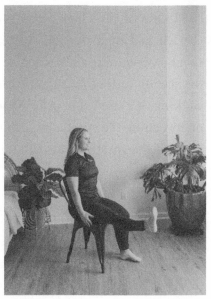

Ankle Dorsiflexion - You can lift both feet at the same time or one foot at a time.

Seated Leg Kicks - Alternate sides

Bowel & Bladder

There are two main types of urinary and bowel symptoms: regular and neurogenic. Regular symptoms include incontinence, urgency, frequency, retention, and hesitation. These are caused by weakness and/or tightness in your pelvic floor. Neurogenic symptoms are caused by miscommunication in the nerves running from the bladder and bowels to the spinal cord to the brain. Physical therapy can have a positive effect on bowel and bladder function through strengthening and stretching the pelvic floor muscles and breathing exercises. Neurogenic bladder is often treated through medication, catheterization, or surgery.

Here's how to differentiate between these symptoms:

- **Incontinence:** Loss of control; severity can range from mild leaking to no control at all.

- **Urgency:** An unexpected need to urinate or have a bowel movement right away.

- **Frequency:** Frequent urges to urinate or have a bowel movement, resulting in going to the bathroom much more than what is typical for your average day.

- **Hesitancy:** Difficulty starting to urinate (or sustaining a steady stream) or have a bowel movement.

- **Retention:** Inability to fully empty your bowels or bladder.

- **Neurogenic Bladder:** When the bladder is spastic, it causes an overactive bladder. When the bladder is flaccid, it causes an underactive bladder. Symptoms include hesitancy, the sensation of incomplete emptying, straining to void, and recurrent infections.

- **Overactive Bladder:** A subtype of neurogenic bladder causing little or no control over emptying your bowel or bladder due to spasticity of the bladder can sometimes be present with urge incontinence.

Some of the symptoms on the list can occur due to a weak and/or tight pelvic floor. The best exercises for symptom management depend on your pelvic floor's strength and flexibility, so it's important to work with a pelvic floor physical therapist to determine the best course of action. Some of my favorite exercises are Kegels to strengthen the pelvic floor, bridging to strengthen the glutes, diaphragmatic breathing to strengthen our belly and core, and the butterfly stretch to stretch our pelvic floor and inner thighs. Core strengthening exercises are also beneficial for improving bladder and bowel control. One of my favorite core exercises is the seated ab lean back. MSing Link member and 1:1 client, Cindy, noticed reduced incontinence and more control in her urination and bowel movements after adding this exercise to her routine.

For more information on exercises and strategies to manage urinary and bowel symptoms, contact a pelvic floor physical therapist.

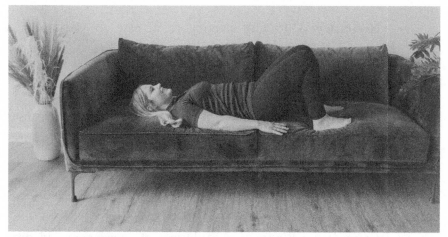

Bridging pt. 1 - Lay flat with knees bent

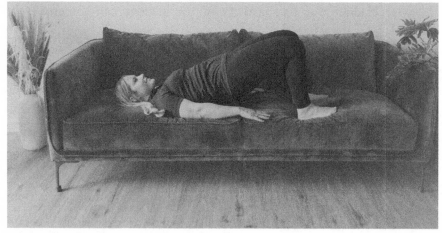

Bridging pt. 2 - Lift your bottom

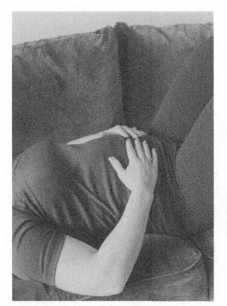

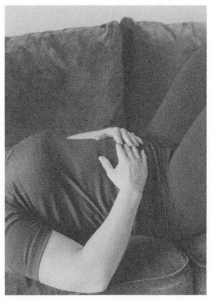

Diaphragmatic Breathing pt. 1 - Inhale as your belly extends out

Diaphragmatic Breathing pt. 2 - Exhale as your belly flattens

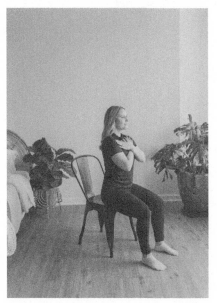

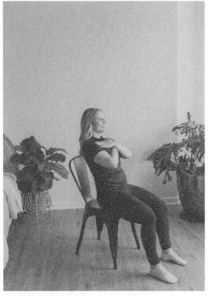

Ab Lean Back pt 1. - Sit up tall with a flat back

Ab Lean Back pt. 2 - Hinge backward while keeping your back flat.

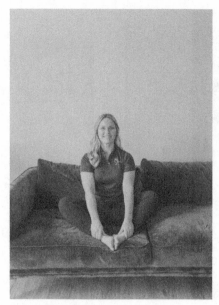

Butterfly Stretch pt. 1 - Let your knees fall open

KEY TAKEAWAYS

1. A primary symptom is caused by the disease process of multiple sclerosis.

2. A secondary symptom is caused by a trigger, like exercise, lack of sleep, stress, an infection, etc.

3. There are many strategies you can implement to reduce invisible symptoms of MS.

4. Have hope! You have more control than you think!

RESOURCES

- To get a pdf & video demonstration of each exercise shown in this book, head to: https://www.doctorgretchenhawley.com/bookpdf

The MSing Link podcast episodes:

- Episode No. 5, "A Solution For Heat & Cold Sensitivity"
- Episode No. 29, "Exercises For Fatigue"
- Episode No. 47, "Pelvic Floor Physical Therapy w/ Dr. Carina Siracusa"
- Episode No. 81, "What is Spasticity & How to Reduce It"
- Episode No. 87, "Sensory Symptoms vs. Motor Symptoms of MS"
- Episode No. 123, "Foot Drop 101"

CHAPTER 3

Neuroplasticity: How and Why You Can Gain Strength ... Even With a Progressive Disease

It's easy to doubt exercise's effectiveness since MS is a progressive disease, especially if you've exercised before and didn't notice much, or any, improvement. The lack of improvement could be due to several factors such as performing the wrong type of exercise. But it is possible to get stronger, walk better, improve your balance, feel more energy, and so on. I'll outline exactly how to do this throughout this book, but it all starts with neuroplasticity.

> Neuroplasticity is the ability of your brain to strengthen your neural pathways and/or find new neural pathways, regardless of the level of demyelination. It's the reason that someone with a progressive disease like MS can get stronger and reach their goals.

However, it takes consistency and time. To fully believe in your improvement, you must understand the nuances of neuroplasticity.

When I ask my clients, "What must happen for a muscle to move?" Nine times out of 10, they'll say: "I have to flex my muscle." This is a common answer, and they're not wrong, but it's much more than that. Misunderstanding the process of how our brain works with our muscles can often result in exercising in the wrong way, leading to no progress. Two things need to happen for any muscle to move or flex.

First, your brain must understand the required action. This occurs either by a reflex, such as you step on something sharp and reflexively you move your leg, or by an active thought where you tell your brain to move your leg. Let's use the example of bending our knees. Once you tell your brain to bend your knee, the second thing that needs to happen is our brain needs to send that message down several neural pathways leading down to the knee. The third thing that happens is the desired movement, in this case, the knee bends.

Your knee won't bend if your brain doesn't think to bend and/ or if the neural pathways aren't working. The reason this three-part sequence is important is because when you focus on strengthening the neural pathways, this leads to muscle strength. However, when you have MS, the second part of the sequence, the neural pathway, is where the breakdown lies due to demyelination. So, even though you're telling yourself, bend my knee, if your neural pathways aren't strong enough, the muscle can't flex as much or at all. This is where neuroplasticity comes into play.

What is Neuroplasticity?

Neuroplasticity is the brain's ability to get the neural pathways working or find a new neural pathway, regardless of the level of demyelination. This can be accomplished in two ways:

1. **Strengthening the pathways that already exist, but have been weakened.** You'll know that your neural pathways are working if you attempt to move a muscle and it moves. You may notice the movement isn't as easy as it once was, but you do see movement. This means that all three parts of the sequence (brain, neural pathway, muscle) are working, but the neural pathway is struggling to produce a force strong enough to fully move your muscle without resistance. Neuroplasticity is the ability to strengthen this neural pathway, so your muscle gains strength and endurance.

2. **Finding a brand-new neural pathway.** Using the example from above, if you attempt to move your muscle and you see no movement at all, this is a sign that your neural pathways have been demyelinated so much, it's not working at all. Neuroplasticity has the capability to rewire your brain to find new neural pathways for those pathways that have lost their ability to make a muscle move. Every time you attempt to move that muscle, your brain will attempt a new pathway to get from your brain to the muscle. There are millions (or who knows maybe trillions!) of different ways to get from point A (your brain) to point B (your muscle) via neural pathways. The only way to find one that works is by repetition—by practicing the desired movement over and over and over again. Do this even if (especially if) there's no movement in the muscle!

Let's think of it differently so we can fully visualize what our brain is capable of doing. Picture yourself driving to the grocery store. Let's say you always drive the same way from your home to the store. Now, imagine driving to the store and there is a roadblock, causing you to return home and try an alternate route. That route, too, has a roadblock, so you turn around and go back home then attempt a different route. You'll repeat this until you find a way to get to the store (or maybe you'll just order groceries from Instacart, but that's not the point here!). Once you arrive at the store, even if the trip was rocky and uneven, you now know this back road option is available and you'll continue to use it moving forward since your preferred route is closed. This road may have started bumpy, however, the more you travel this path, the smoother and easier the trip becomes.

> Simply practicing the right type of movements over and over again will strengthen the pathway from your brain to your muscle, which in turn strengthens your muscles.

Don't give up! Every repetition matters, even if there is little to no movement in the exercise you're practicing.

How Long Does Neuroplasticity Take?

Neuroplasticity can happen for anyone with MS regardless of your level of disability or the length of time you've had MS. I've had clients who have had MS for 37-plus years and they were able to strengthen their muscles, walk better (with less foot drag and tripping) and feel more confident. If you have demyelination from MS, and if you have neural pathways that aren't working, that's not the end of the game for you. It doesn't mean that you can't get stronger. Use the strategies in this book to create a plan of attack. You'll start to see and feel an improvement over time.

Generally speaking, strengthening an existing neural pathway doesn't take as long as finding a brand new neural pathway. At this time, no research provides a protocol for neuroplasticity. Meaning, no guide says, "repeat each of your desired movements 50 times per day for 12 weeks and that's when you'll start to see improvements in your strength and mobility." I've had some clients who will do these repetitions over and over and over again, and truly within a few days, they notice their knee bending has improved. Many of my clients notice improvements in three months, six months or 12 months. Remember,

MS is the snowflake disease, but our brains are different, too. Many factors play a role in how quickly clients find or create new neural pathways. Some we can control, others we can't control. This takes a lot of resilience. Your brain can find a brand new neural pathway, but it might require performing that movement or multiple movements for a year, or a year and a half, without seeing results. It's important not to associate the amount of movement with success, rather, associate the amount of effort you put into each exercise with success. This way, it's easier to stay consistent for the long haul and you won't feel like a failure. More effort = more opportunities for neuroplasticity.

Another thing doctors don't know, yet, is the effectiveness of neuroplasticity in spinal lesions. There is a lot of research on the effectiveness of neuroplasticity for people with brain lesions, including but not limited to Dr. Dominika Ksiazek-Winiarek from RUSH Medical College study titled "Neural Plasticity in Multiple Sclerosis: The Functional and Molecular Background." But there is little to no research on neuroplasticity for people with spinal lesions. It's been a life goal of mine to find this answer. In my medical journal research and from conversations with MS neurologists and researchers, the assumption is this: Since neuroplasticity occurs in those with brain lesions, it likely occurs in those with spinal lesions. Additionally, there's no negative side effect to exercising with the goal of seeing neuroplastic changes if you have spinal lesions. Let's do the best and worst-case scenario for a second. In the worst-case scenario, exercising doesn't result in physical improvements. But you reap the benefits of exercise such as feeling happy due to the surge of feel-good hormones (endorphins) released in your body and improved heart and brain health. In the best-case scenario, exercising improves mobility, increases strength and inspires engagement in new and old activities.

Ways to Activate Neuroplasticity

It's exciting that neuroplasticity is available to us, but it's even more exciting to increase the likelihood of it happening! I've outlined five of the most widely known concepts to get neuroplasticity working.

1. **Focused attention:** The more focus on an exercise or activity, the more likely you are to see improvements due to neuroplastic changes. With focused attention, you can create up to 1.8 million new connections per second. So, when you're exercising, avoid multitasking, including thinking about your next meal or completing the mile-long list of errands. Pay attention to the exercise, so your brain can figure out how to make the desired movement happen.

2. **Alertness:** Play a game to stimulate your mind and focus your attention. Turn the exercise into a game and lift your leg high enough to tap your hand. Or do an exercise for the duration of the chorus of your favorite song. Maybe toss a ball back and forth with a friend or by yourself while maintaining a good sitting or standing posture! Take your brain off autopilot to stay alert.

3. **Urgency:** The more urgent a task, the more likely you'll see neuroplastic changes. A great way to build urgency into your exercises is to create some level of consequence. For example, if you're practicing balance, stand on an uneven surface with the consequence of stepping off the surface. Or, you could score yourself, with the consequence being "losing" the game. Urgency works well for people who are competitive with themselves, but it can work for everyone. Find a way to build urgency into your movements.

4. **Novelty:** One simple way to get your brain to pay attention is to try something new. For example, try writing with your non-dominant hand. This will take much more focus and alertness than writing with your dominant hand. Making the brain try new activities drives neurologic change!

Setting these four factors in place (Focused Attention, Alertness, Urgency, and Novelty) creates the chemical conditions in the brain for neuroplasticity to happen. Once this occurs, the brain can begin to rewire itself. The more we prime our brain in this way, the more likely we are to see improvements in our mobility at a quicker rate. You can use one or a few of these factors in combination with your exercises or you can use them during your break. For example, after you complete one set of each of your exercises, attempt to write your name with your non-dominant hand. Or, take a break to play a one-minute game of tossing a ball, or any game that makes you alert. Or between each set of exercises, practice a balance exercise where the consequence is to avoid stepping off an uneven surface. Always be safe with these games, you don't want to put yourself in a position where you lose your balance, fall, or injure yourself.

5. **Salience:** The more meaningful the activity is, the more likely your brain will create neuroplastic changes. The easiest way to accomplish this is to create meaning for each exercise. For example, "This marching exercise will help me lift my leg higher, which means I won't trip as often during my walks with my husband and two kids." Or "This balance exercise will allow me to bend down to the floor to pick up the dog food bowl and feed my dog without falling over." Take time to think about your goals and how these exercises can help you reach them.

Exercise Guidelines to Increase Neuroplasticity in MS

1. **Aim for almost-perfect quality:** Having almost-perfect quality is important. Your brain will strengthen the pathway for the movement you repeat. If repetitions are performed with poor form, your neural pathways will remember what you practiced and strengthen those pathways. This could significantly impact your quality of

movement and may cause unsteadiness and falls. Good quality = good neural pathways. You'll know if you're performing good quality exercises when you see the ideal movement. For example, sitting in a chair with both feet on the ground. Lift your toes and forefoot up, your foot should appear to be straight, not angled with one side of your foot rolling inward or outward. Similarly, when lifting your leg, your leg should lift straight up without your knee falling inward or outward.

2. **Repeat, repeat, repeat:** To increase your odds of strengthening or finding a successful pathway, you must practice consistently. The goal for every exercise is to perform many good quality repetitions. The number of times you practice is equivalent to the number of times your brain attempts to find that pathway. Now, you may be thinking, "How am I supposed to do as many repetitions as I can but also have good quality? I'm going to get tired!" You're right. And this point brings me to my next guideline.

3. **Rest!:** Take as many breaks as needed. When you have MS, the goal shouldn't be to perform each exercise 10 times, in sets of three, like we were taught growing up. You can set a goal of 30 good-quality repetitions, but that may take seven sets of various repetitions, assuming you're fatigued as you complete more repetitions. For example, your first set is 10, but due to fatigue, your second set might be six. Your third and fourth sets may be four repetitions. Your fifth and six sets could be three repetitions. And that's okay! Neuroplasticity doesn't require a bunch of exercises all at once, but it does need the cumulative amount to be a high number.

4. **Choose a duration:** Would you believe me if I told you research suggests exercise is equally effective if you exercise throughout the day or all at once? It's true. Professor Marie Murphy of Ulster University found this to be true in her 2019 meta-analytic review. This means if you have the time and preference to exercise for 20 to 60 minutes all at once, go for it! However, if you don't have

the time, energy level, or preference to exercise all at once, you'll still benefit from fitting it in throughout the day. One idea is to associate breaks with one exercise. This way, you can pick an exercise and perform good quality repetitions, within five minutes, while taking rest breaks. Then, later in the day, do the same thing but with a different exercise. By the end of the day, you will have completed four to seven exercises.

5. **Exercise in different settings:** Research shows you're more likely to feel and see improvements in various situations and environments (i.e. you're walking better in your home as well as in the grocery store), if you practice exercising in multiple locations. One easy way to do this is to practice exercises in different rooms within your home. Perhaps one day, you exercise in the kitchen. Then, the next day, exercise in the bedroom. The following day, the living room, and so on. Take this even further by practicing some of your exercises outdoors (i.e. walking, seated exercises sitting on a rollator, etc.). You could also do your exercises in your car, at a friend's house and at work. Get creative!

One of my MSing Link members and clients, Diane, had a goal to improve her strength when standing up, while also trying to "plop" down less often. I suggested specific exercises to strengthen her leg and core muscles, in addition to practicing standing up from a chair and sitting back down with control. She was consistent with her exercises and did a phenomenal job. Her husband attended a session and said, "Dr. Gretchen, I don't know what magic you're doing in this clinic, but Diane can stand up and sit down perfectly when she is here with you, but as soon as we get home, she can't do it." As soon as he said that, I remembered the benefits of exercising in different settings. We immediately started performing the exercises in other rooms within the PT clinic, the lobby, other offices in the building, and even outside on a bench. Within one month, she was able to perform this movement at home with much more control and strength. Both Diane and her husband were extremely happy.

6. **Choose a plan:** According to the National MS Society, 150 minutes per week is the desired amount of exercise to reap the benefits. Further, MS exercise guidelines from the National Center on Health, Physical Activity, and Disability (NCHPAD) suggest people with MS should exercise five to six days per week. This means exercising five days a week for 30 minutes per day. Or, three days a week for 50 minutes. And so on. This can be cumulative or all at once. To take this a step further, research suggests switching up the type of exercise and the order of your exercises. Don't always start and end with the same exercises. Mix it up!

7. **Do cardio first:** A study called "Exercise-Induced Neuroplasticity" led by researcher Jenin El-Sayes from McMaster University in Ontario, Canada found that performing cardio exercises before functional strengthening exercises will prime your brain for neuroplasticity. Meaning, you're even more likely to find and strengthen neural pathways if you do cardio exercise first! This is newer research (multiple studies published in 2018, 2019 and 2020), so we don't know the exact guidelines, yet. No protocol says cardio needs to be X minutes long at Y intensity to be effective. I guide my clients to perform any amount of cardio they can tolerate. I suggest using your arms for cardio instead of your legs. This way, you won't exhaust your legs before the leg strengthening exercises. Some of my favorite cardio movements are sitting up tall with good posture while swinging your arms next to your body (as if you're running) for one minute. Then, do overhead jumping jacks with just your arms for one minute and end with punching your arms forward for one minute. This will get your heart rate up in no time.

KEY TAKEAWAYS

1. Neuroplasticity is the ability of our brain to strengthen neural pathways and find new neural pathways.

2. Strong neural pathways lead to strong muscles and improved mobility.

3. Neuroplasticity can happen for anyone with MS regardless of your level of disability or the length of time you've had the disease.

4. There are specific ways to exercise to activate neuroplasticity and make it more likely to occur faster.

5. If you attempt to move a body part (i.e. your ankle) and it doesn't move, this is not an excuse to skip the exercise, instead it's a reason to prioritize that particular exercise. Give your brain a chance to find a new neural pathway by repeating the exercise, even with no movement. One repetition equals one bout of effort.

6. Have hope! Research shows it's possible!

RESOURCES

The MSing Link podcast episodes:

- Episode No. 3, "What is Neuroplasticity?"
- Episode No. 96, "How Long Does Neuroplasticity Take?"
- Episode No. 99, "Aerobic Exercise & Neuroplasticity"

CHAPTER 4

Move Your Body: 10 Exercises to Improve Your Overall Strength and Conditioning

When I ask my clients what types of exercises exist, the most common answer is aerobic exercises, strengthening exercises, and possibly stretching. How would you feel if I told you there are actually more than 10 types of exercises and that when you have MS, it's integral to incorporate a combination of at least six types of exercises? It's true! Let's dive in:

Strengthening: If you want to get stronger, you must perform some form of strength training. This can be referred to as weight training, using any type of weight including dumbbells, barbells, weighted balls, etc. Or resistance training with resistance bands, or bodyweight training with no equipment. You can also strengthen your muscles on machines at the gym, as well as aerobic machines like a stationary and recumbent bike and an elliptical machine. The goal of strength training is to strengthen muscles, sometimes individually and sometimes in multiple muscle groups at a time. It also can help strengthen joints and bones.

With MS, it's extremely important to perform functional strengthening exercises to improve walking, climbing stairs, standing up from a low surface, sitting down without plopping, and getting into and out of your car. More on this in the next chapter. That's right, it's important enough to have its own chapter! Examples of functional strengthening include heel raises, marching, and hamstring curls.

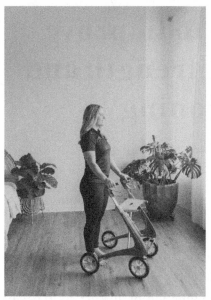 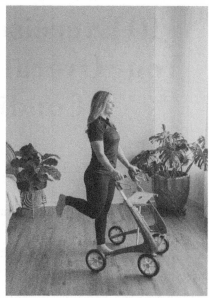

Hamstring Curl pt. 1 - Stand up tall

Hamstring Curl pt. 2 - Bend your knee as much as possible, even if it's a few centimeters.

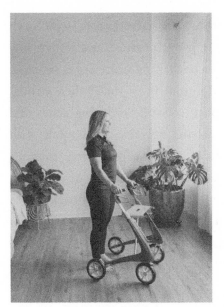

Heel Raises pt. 1 - Stand up tall

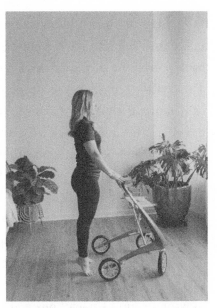

Heel Raises pt. 2 - Raise your heels off the floor

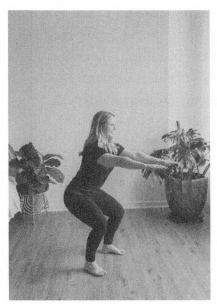

Squats - Pretend to sit down in a chair while keeping your arms and shoulders forward to keep yourself steady.

Let's not forget about the importance of a strong core, which can make walking and movement easier, improve posture, and reduce low back pain. One of my favorite core strengthening exercises is bracing. This will strengthen the deepest abdominal layer that, when strong, can improve walking, balance, and posture while reducing aches and pains in the lower back. To perform this exercise, sit up tall with your hips and back touching the back of a chair. From here, use your abdominal muscles to push your lower back into the back of the chair. There shouldn't be any space between the chair and your back. Once there, hold for up to 10 seconds then release and repeat. Once you're a pro at this exercise, you can progress by trying it while sitting at the edge of your chair, standing against a wall, and standing away from the wall. The most advanced version is to perform this exercise while moving around throughout your day.

Another favorite core exercise of mine is the ab lean back. To practice this, sit up tall at the edge of your chair, brace your abdominal muscles using the technique above, and hinge backward toward the back of the chair while keeping your back flat. Your arms can be straight out in front of you (this is the easiest position), or crossed over your chest (this is the hardest version). Hold for up to three seconds, then return to the start position and repeat.

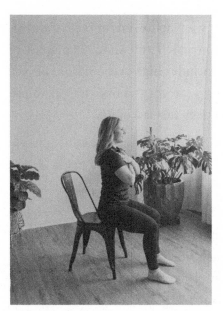

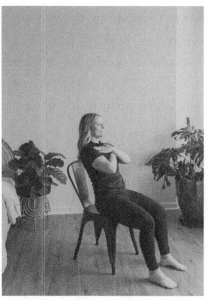

Ab Lean Back pt 1. - Sit up tall with a flat back

Ab Lean Back pt. 2 - Hinge backward while keeping your back flat; you should mostly feel this in your abdomen. If you feel it in your hip flexors, don't hinge back as far.

Endurance: To use your muscles for a longer time, such as walking a longer distance or maintaining a tall posture, you must train your muscles for endurance. Endurance training is similar to strengthening, but instead of splitting up the repetitions into many different sets, you want to practice as many repetitions as you can at one time. Essentially, this trains the body to use that muscle for a longer period of time. For example, doing 40 repetitions will take longer than doing 10 repetitions. Therefore, if you continually practice 40 repetitions, you'll have more endurance. Similarly, if your goal is to maintain good posture, seated or standing, for a longer time then you should practice sitting or standing with good posture for as long as you can. Practicing holding a good posture for three to five minutes will improve endurance more than holding good posture for one minute, three to five times. This is challenging and often requires improved strength first, so slowly work your way up to endurance training, instead of pushing yourself to do too much too soon. Examples of functional endurance movements include high repetitions of the exercises listed in the "strengthening" category above. For example, you could perform 25 marching exercises instead of 10.

Stretching: This is one of the best ways to reduce muscle tightness in addition to other muscle relaxing techniques, such as massage and muscle rolling. There are three types of stretches:

- **Static:** Hold a stretch for longer periods of time, typically 20 to 30 seconds. For the most effective stretching, perform this two to four times on each side. For example, stretch your right hamstring two to four times with a 20 to 30-second hold each time. Repeat on your left side.

- **Dynamic:** Hold a stretch for shorter durations, typically two to three seconds. For the most effective stretching, perform each stretch 20 to 30 times. For example, get into a position where you feel your hamstring stretching and hold it for two to three seconds, then back off to release the stretch. After one to two seconds, stretch again, hold for two to three seconds, and back off. Repeat 20 to 30 times on each side.

- **Prolonged static:** Hold a stretch for a prolonged period, typically five to seven minutes. Perform this once on each side or both sides at the same time. You should be fully relaxed to get the most out of the stretch. Research shows that both static and dynamic stretching are equally effective, and prolonged static stretching is best for spastic muscles (according to Dr. Tamis Pin from University of Melbourne and other researchers). This is why I encourage my clients to try both and see which one feels best. If neither feels better than the other, pick whichever one feels easier to implement into your day.

There are numerous effective positions you can stretch in such as standing, sitting, lying down, etc. I prefer seated stretches because people sit most of the day. This helps release muscle tightness and tension that builds up the longer you're in one position. The reason these are functional is because they're positions we often find ourselves in throughout the day.

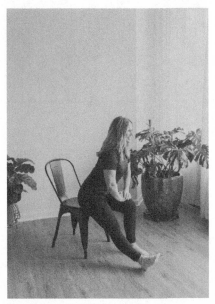

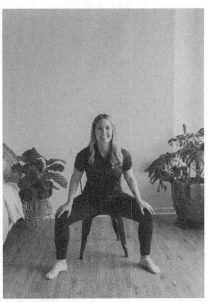

Hamstring Stretch - Keep one knee as straight as possible and hinge forward. You can also do this stretch standing. You should feel this stretch in the back of your thigh and knee.

Inner Thigh Stretch - You should feel this stretch in your inner thighs.

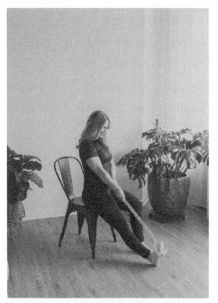

Calf Stretch - Use a non-stretchy item to pull your toes and forefoot toward you; you should feel this stretch in the back of your lower leg.

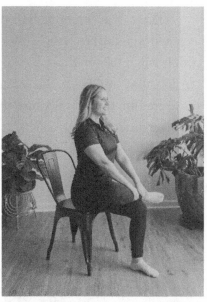

Figure 4 Stretch - Place one ankle on the opposite lower leg; sit up tall to feel a stretch in the outer hip.

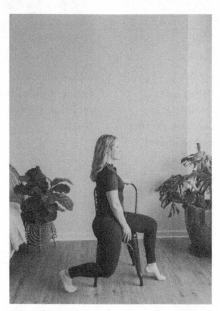

Hip Flexor Stretch - You should feel this stretch in the front of your hip and/or front of your thigh.

Balance: This is the ability to distribute your weight to stand or move without falling, or recover if you trip. It requires the coordination of several parts of the body, including the central nervous system, inner ear/vestibular, eyes, muscles, bones, and joints. We need balance when we're seated and standing. The two main types of balance are static, a.k.a. stationary, no movement such as sitting up tall or standing tall; and dynamic, a.k.a. moving balance such as reaching into your closet, reaching into the dishwasher, walking, etc. Examples of functional balance include lateral weight shifting, staggered stance weight shifting, and single-leg stance balance. You can practice these while holding onto a mobility aid or a steady surface for more stability.

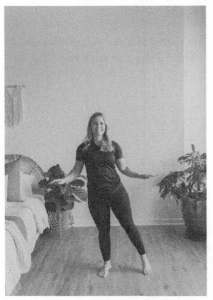 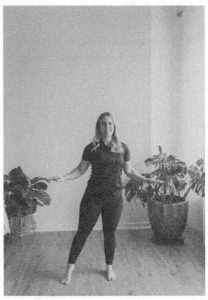

Lateral Weight Shifting pt. 1 - Shift weight to your right side

Lateral Weight Shifting pt. 2 - Shift weight to your left side

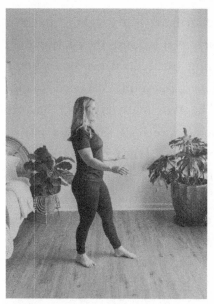

Staggered Stance Weight Shift pt. 1 - Shift weight to your back leg

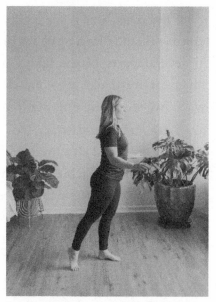

Staggered Stance Weight Shift pt. 2 - Shift weight to your front leg

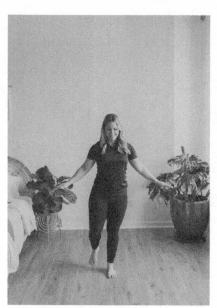

Single Leg Stance - Lift one leg off the floor in any way you can: bend your knee, raise your leg out to the side, hang off of a step, etc.

Coordination: Do you ever feel like you look drunk when you're walking? If so, it's probably due to poor coordination. Your feet aren't landing where you want them to. Sometimes this occurs due to weak or tight muscles, but other times it's strictly due to a lack of coordination. This can be dangerous because it often results in hitting your feet together or tripping over your feet. Poor coordination can also occur in the upper body, which often results in difficulty placing your hand and fingers where you want them to go.

My favorite example of a coordination exercise is to practice taking a single step forward, but tapping your heel on a quarter. Return to the start position and repeat. This trains your brain to place your heel in a specific location rather than wherever your heel lands. For the upper body, practice reaching forward and touching a quarter that is placed on a table in front of you, then touching the same finger to your nose. Repeat this movement.

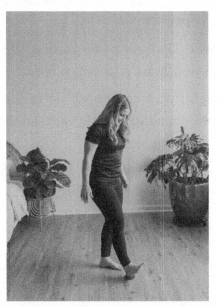

Cone/Quarter Tap - Attempt to lift your leg and tap the item with your heel. Make sure you're standing close enough to the item so you're not reaching too far in front of you to tap the item.

Aerobic exercise: As you know from the previous chapter, one benefit of aerobic exercise is that it primes the brain for neuroplasticity when it's performed before functional strengthening exercises. However, aerobic exercise is also important for heart and brain health! The goal of aerobic exercise is to increase your heart rate. You can use machines such as a treadmill, elliptical, or bike to accomplish this, or your body weight. My favorite way to perform aerobic exercise is seated and using only my arms. This way, your legs aren't fatigued when it's time to do leg strengthening exercises.

Here are four ways to make any upper or lower body movement into an aerobic workout:

- **Move faster:** Anytime you move faster, your heart works harder.

- **Aim for bigger movement:** This will slow you down, but since it's challenging to move with full motion, it'll increase your heart rate.

- **Add power:** The more power you put behind each movement, the more your heart rate will increase.

- **Add weight:** With upper body aerobic exercises, hold onto a one to two-pound weight. If you're doing lower body aerobic exercises, add ankle weights.

Examples of seated upper-body aerobic exercises include arm swings, forward punches, and upper body jumping jacks.

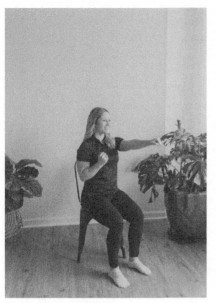

Forward Punches pt. 1

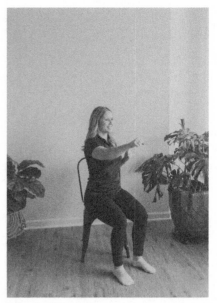

Forward Punches pt. 2

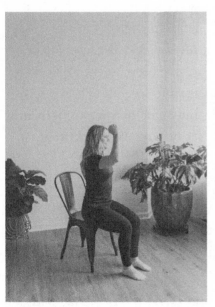

Arm Swing pt. 1

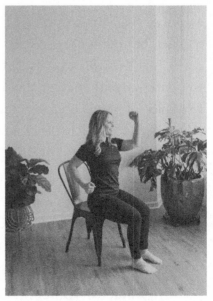

Arm Swing pt. 2

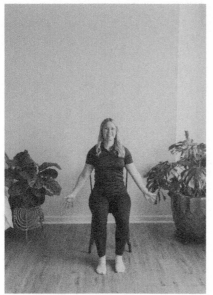
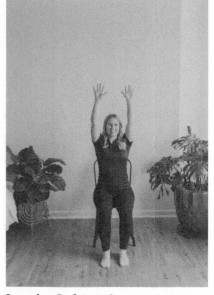

Jumping Jacks pt. 1   **Jumping Jacks pt. 2**

Speed: If your goal is to move faster, practice speed-based exercises. Sometimes speed is reduced due to tight, weak or spastic muscles, but other times it's less than ideal simply because you're not practicing speed. Speed is its own category of exercise, meaning even if you improve your strength and balance, your speed may not improve. Examples of speed exercises include the same as the strengthening exercises, but with a focus of moving faster with each repetition.

Implementing daily movement: Things like getting out of bed, getting dressed, showering, getting the mail, walking to and from the car, cooking, climbing stairs, etc. count, especially if you're low energy or don't have enough time to perform your regular exercise routine. Don't discount the amount of strength and effort it takes to perform these daily movements.

High-intensity interval training (HIIT): Dr. Nadine Patt and her colleagues' research displayed in BMC Neurology (2021) indicate that HIIT is an effective form of exercise for people with multiple sclerosis. The way to achieve HIIT is to go back and forth between a high-intensity exercise and a low-intensity exercise. It can sound scary at first, but anyone can perform this exercise. Make a list of easy and challenging exercises. Your heart rate will increase based on effort. Remember, this will look different for everyone based on strength, tightness, endurance, etc. For example:

High-Intensity Exercise	Low-Intensity Exercise
• Marching	• Arm swings
• Squats	• Forward punches
• Hamstring curl	• Weight shifting

Once you have your list, you're ready to practice. Choose one of the high-intensity exercises and perform it for as long as you can until you get fatigued, typically around 30 seconds to one minute. To get your heart rate up while performing the movement, refer to the aerobic exercise tips above. Once you're done, choose a lower-intensity exercise and perform that until your heart rate comes down but is not fully rested, typically around one to two minutes. Each person requires different interval timing, but use this as a guide and then adjust from there.

Classes: There are various classes that often work with a combination of the exercises covered here. For example, yoga, pilates, tai chi, dance, swimming or aqua aerobics, boxing, rowing, etc. These are great options, but should not replace functional training or any specific training mentioned above. Classes should be an addition to the other forms of exercise you practice.

Fun fact: Newer research in 2022 from my colleague Alexander Ng from Marquette University suggests seated ballroom dancing is an effective form of rehab for people with MS! After learning this, I implemented seated ballroom dance classes in The MSing Link, taught by a physical therapist assistant and ballroom dancer. After four months, my MSing Link members noticed better posture, better walking endurance, and better walking quality. And their cheeks hurt from smiling during class!

> Beware of only performing one type of exercise consistently. It may sound counterintuitive, but focusing on one form of exercise can lead to injuries, pain, and muscular imbalance, even if that exercise focuses on multiple categories like strength, balance, endurance, and flexibility.

This occurs because it's easy for our bodies to use the muscles that are already strong and balanced without focusing on the weakest muscles. Over time, this causes strain on muscles and joints.

For example, my MSing Link client, Sarah, initially came to work with me because she suffered from lower back pain. As an avid yoga student, attending classes 4 to 5 days per week, she didn't do any other form of exercise since yoga covered most bases: strength, stretching, and balance. But as soon as Sarah focused on strengthening specific muscles and dynamic stretching, instead of static stretching, her pain started to dissipate. The same situation occurred with Amanda, another client. She solely focused on weight training. Over time, Amanda developed hip and knee pain, which caused her to have foot drop, and hip-swing while walking. Once she incorporated stretching, endurance training, and balance training, her pain decreased, allowing her to walk with better quality for a longer time.

Which Exercise is Right For You?

The types of exercise in your routine depend on your symptoms and goals. For example, if you have any goal related to walking (i.e. less tripping, walking longer distances, less hip-swinging, etc.) you should incorporate strength training, stretching, balance, endurance, coordination, and speed for your legs. If the goal is to improve your posture, focus on strengthening, stretching, endurance, balance, and implementation for your core, back, and shoulders.

There are several exercises you can do for each category, based on your symptoms, but let's call out the elephant in the room, that's a LOT of exercises! Don't worry, you don't need to perform all of them in your routine at first. Prioritize exercises based on your dominant symptoms. Ask yourself what top three symptoms are causing the biggest disruption in my day? From there, choose exercises associated with those symptoms. If you can't tell, work with an MS-specialized or neuro-specialized physical therapist to determine which movements should be prioritized.

Once you know which categories you'll prioritize, pick which exercises you'll do. This step is especially important for people with packed schedules, but want to get the biggest bang for the buck from their workout.

> I encourage my clients to start with challenging exercises first because they identify weak muscles. When you focus on the weakest muscles first, you'll see a faster improvement, than if you start with stronger muscles.

Another option is to choose easy exercises. If they're easier, you're more likely to do them consistently, and see results. Once you're more consistent, add in more difficult exercises.

An ideal exercise routine consists of three or four types of exercise each day. For example, you could combine:

- three strengthening exercises
- one to two balance exercises
- one coordination exercise
- two to three stretches

> Note: Depending on the exercise, this will take about 30 minutes.

On a different day, you can combine:

- five minutes of aerobic/cardio (upper body only, lower body only, or both)
- two strengthening exercises
- two endurance exercises
- two speed exercises

> Note: Depending on the exercise, this will take about 30 minutes.

BONUS TIP: If the goal is to improve balance, practice walking slowly with exaggerated movements to and from the bathroom. This type of practice will train your brain to understand your desire to improve strength and balance while exercising and in real life situations throughout the day.

Here is an example of an exercise routine you could follow for several weeks or months if you aim to improve your walking. This includes a combination of strength, cardio, and balance training in addition to stretching, coordination, and a class. The routine below is assuming that you have the time and energy to exercise for six days per week, however, if you don't, simply choose the exercises associated with just one column.

The exercises listed can be performed all at once, taking about 20-30 minutes, or throughout the day in small chunks of time, about five minutes or less. You can implement each exercise for up to 30 good-quality repetitions using the information you've learned earlier in this book. Remember you can take as many breaks as you need during each exercise.

Exercise Routine Example		
MONDAY WEDNESDAY FRIDAY	TUESDAY, THURSDAY	SATURDAY
Cardio (3-5 minutes)	Cardio (3-5 minutes)	Yoga Class, or
Leg Kicks	Ab Lean Back	Go for a walk, or
Marching	Squats	Swim/Aqua Aerobic Class, or
Ankle Dorsiflexion	Lateral Weight Shifting	any form of movement for 20 minutes
Hamstring Stretch	Cone Taps	

Use the pictures presented in this book as a guide.

KEY TAKEAWAYS

1. There are 10 types of exercise: strengthening, endurance, stretching, balance, coordination, aerobic, speed, classes, implementation, and HIIT.

2. Your exercise routine should include at least six types of exercises throughout the week.

3. Focusing on one form of exercise can often lead to injuries, pain, and muscular imbalance, even if that exercise focuses on multiple categories like strength, balance, endurance, and flexibility.

4. Implementing exercises throughout the day is a great way to train your brain to understand that this way of moving is your new norm!

5. Have hope! You can do this!

RESOURCES

- To get a pdf & video demonstration of each exercise shown in this book, head to: https://www.doctorgretchenhawley.com/bookpdf

- The MSing Link podcast episode No. 69, "5 Types of Exercise - Are You Choosing The Right One?"

CHAPTER 5

The RIGHT Way to Exercise with MS

As you know by now, all exercises are *not* created equal! If your goal is to gain strength, but you aren't working toward improved mobility or making your day-to-day actions easier and less fatiguing, then traditional strengthening exercises are helpful. However, if you're looking to improve your function throughout the day, trip/fall less, and improve your endurance/stamina, research shows you must exercise differently.

Have you ever noticed when you follow an exercise program or a physical therapy routine, you get stronger, but your walking doesn't get any easier? Or do you feel stronger, but climbing stairs is just as challenging? Or maybe your balance exercises are improving, but you're still tripping and falling? This can be an eye-opening realization that not all exercises are created equal! The likely culprit causing no improvement in your day-to-day function isn't the exercise you're doing, it's the exercise you're *not* doing.

I consider "regular" exercise or "traditional" physical therapy exercises to be general exercise. The other type, functional exercise, is one that will help you not only improve strength and balance, but it will also improve day-to-day functions like walking, getting in and out of bed, climbing stairs, standing up from low surfaces, etc.

There are several steps in determining the best functional exercises for you, starting with choosing one or more goals you're working toward, then breaking down that goal/activity into as many movements as possible. Those movements should be part of your daily exercise routine.

If you're wondering if you are performing functional exercises or not then there are a few questions you can ask yourself:

Are the exercises I'm doing in the same position as my goal? For example, if your goal is to walk longer distances, are the majority of your exercises done in a standing position? After all, when you're walking, you're standing! If the answer is no, then it may be time to re-evaluate the exercises.

Am I spending a lot of time exercising on a recumbent bicycle? Bicycles, recumbent or otherwise, are a great form of exercise for cardio and leg strengthening, however, they are only functional if you have a goal of biking better or longer. But since biking is performed seated, it isn't a functional exercise for goals in a standing position, such as improving your walking or stair climbing. You may get stronger legs and improved cardiovascular endurance but see no gains in walking. Too often, my clients focus on biking longer and resistance building thinking it'll improve their walking ability when in reality, it doesn't.

Am I using weights, machines, or resistance bands? These can be great additions to make exercise more challenging down the road, but all functional exercises should start off without any resistance or added weight, so you can use the proper muscles without overcompensating with stronger muscles.

Here's why performing exercises in a functional position matters: With MS, your brain, neural pathways, and muscles don't have the same carryover as someone without MS. So, you might have full strength seated on a bike or lying on your back or your side, but when you go to stand up, that strength is nonexistent.

This often occurs with general orthopedic physical therapy exercises. You may perform some exercises lying on a treatment table like the straight leg raise, clamshell, and bridging, and build up to full strength in your leg muscles. While these exercises are very functional for lying down movements such as moving around in bed, the brain, neural pathways, and muscles don't have the same carryover, meaning you likely won't notice improved strength while standing or walking.

Arlene, one of my physical therapy clients with MS, participated in traditional physical therapy in hopes of improving her walking quality and walking longer distances. A typical session included exercises such as riding a recumbent bicycle and general strengthening exercises. Over time, Arlene could bike longer and with higher resistance (i.e. biking for 30 minutes at resistance level five), and she improved her strength with the exercises. But there was no difference in her walking, which was the main goal.

Why did this happen?

> Someone who has MS does not have the same muscular carryover as someone without MS, meaning you may notice improved strength when sitting, but not standing or walking.

While Arlene improved to the point of full strength in her legs when sitting on a bike and lying on a treatment table, when she stood up, that strength was non-existent. Her brain and neural pathways didn't understand that the strength gained should be applied in all positions, not just the exercise position. This is a very typical experience for someone with MS who isn't performing functional exercises.

After several months of working with me utilizing the concepts of neuroplasticity and functional exercise, Arlene felt stronger, empowered, and confident with her newfound independence with walking.

One easy way to ensure you're performing a functional exercise is to do the movement in the same position as your goal. For example, if you want to have less difficulty getting into and out of a car, then replicate this movement by practicing moving your legs up and over an object from a seated position, ideally in a car, but any chair will do. If you normally get into a car from a standing position, then you'd do the same exercise while standing. A quick side note: One helpful tool to stay balanced while getting into a car is a car cane. I'll link to this in the resources page at the back of the book.

And for improved strength when standing up from the ground, practice moving from kneeling to standing. If you want to trip less, practice bending your knee and lifting your leg higher while standing. I know you may be thinking: "This sounds great, but my MS has caused weakness that won't allow me to perform exercises in these positions." Stay with me. I'll explain how this is doable for everyone.

The second way to ensure you're performing functional exercise is to break down your goal into as many micro movements as possible and practice those movements. Let's stick with the example of improving the quality of your walking.

Walking is many movements put together for one swift movement. I want you to visualize with me for a second. Picture yourself standing with your feet shoulder width apart. One foot is forward and the opposite foot is behind it, in a staggered position. Now, to take one single step forward, perform these movements:

1. Shift your weight forward onto the front leg.

2. Bend your back knee so your heel comes closer to your buttock.

3. Lift your ankle and toes up, which will reduce foot drop.

4. Bring your knee up towards the ceiling.

5. Straighten your knee.

6. Put your heel down.

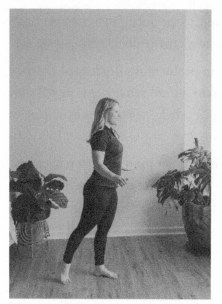

Step 1 - Shift Weight Forward

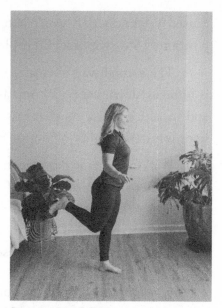

Step 2 - Bend Knee

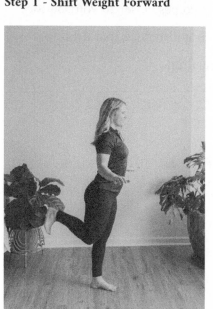

Step 3 - Lift Toes

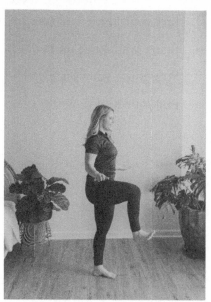

Step 4 - Bring Knee Forward

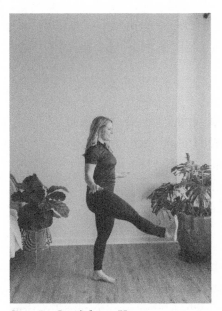
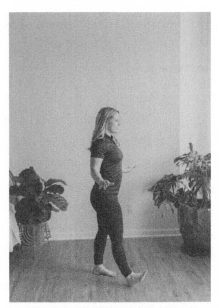

Step 5 - Straighten Knee   **Step 6 - Place Heel Down**

Note: While one leg is moving forward, you are standing on one leg. Whether you were using an assistive device or not, you were still standing on one leg, leading to one final step:

7.   Balance on one leg, with or without a mobility aid.

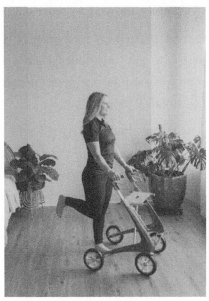

In the pictures shown above, I'm exaggerating every movement. You don't have to lift your leg that high to reap the benefits. Any movement will work.

> Walking consists of seven different movements, and these can be turned into seven different exercises. If the goal is to improve walking quality and/or endurance, you shouldn't focus solely on walking. You must practice these seven functional movements, too.

For example, perform each of these exercises, or just a few, for 10 repetitions each. These are the strengthening components needed to improve walking. Other components include arm swing, coordination, core strength and flexibility in your hamstrings, quadriceps, and ankle.

You might find that some of those movements (above) are somewhat easier for you and maybe others are more challenging. If ANY of those movements are difficult, it can throw off your walking. Therefore, whether you add one exercise or all seven, any of these will help improve your walking in addition to practicing walking as a whole.

Let's take it one step further. Not only do we now know that we should break down our goal into several movements in addition to exercising in the same position as our goal, but what do we do if it's too challenging? Let's break it down.

One of those seven movements that we broke down was bringing your knee up toward the ceiling—I call this a marching exercise. You can practice marching in a standing position, of course, which is going to be the most functional position since when we walk, we're in a standing position. However, at first, that might be too challenging for you. So, you can choose to practice marching in a different position, like seated, reclined, lying on your back, or lying on your side. Photos of these exercise positions can be found in the next chapter.

The idea is to pick a position that allows you to do several good-quality repetitions. When you get stronger, you can change to a more functional position, eventually working your way to a standing position. This strategy is extremely helpful for neuroplasticity because the easier the exercise is, the more repetitions you'll be able to do.

> The more repetitions you can do, the more opportunities you're giving your brain to strengthen that neural pathway, which is the whole point!

What is The BEST Functional Exercise For MS?

Anytime I'm asked what the BEST functional exercise is, my answer is, "do the thing that's hard." The absolute best way to make sure you're including functional exercises into your routine is to physically put yourself in the position of the goal you're trying to achieve. Make it easier at first, then work your way up to doing the full movement. For example, if you're struggling standing up from low surfaces like the toilet or a chair or bench, practice standing up from low surfaces! However, make sure your surface is manageable so you can do it successfully. This often requires picking a higher surface, at first. Then, as you get stronger, slowly pick lower surfaces to stand up from. Repeat this as an exercise.

Let's break down the function/activity of standing up into functional exercises. Here's what's required:

1. Sit up tall.

2. Scoot forward.

3. Separate your feet and your knees into a wide stance.

4. Bend your knees.

5. Hinge forward.

6. Stand up.

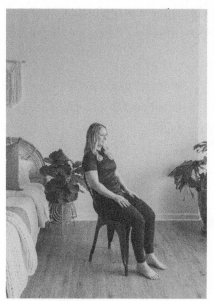

Start Position

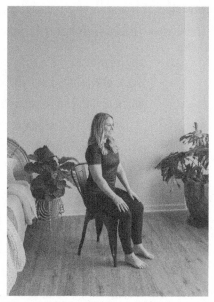

Step 1- Sit Up Tall

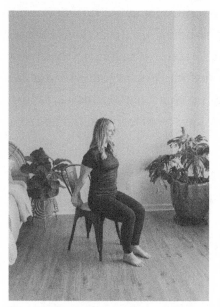

Step 2 - Scoot Forward

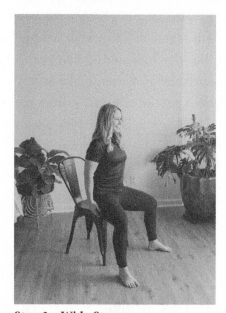

Step 3 - Wide Stance

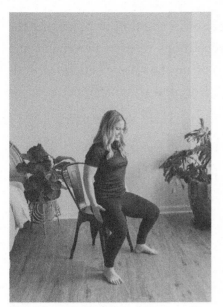

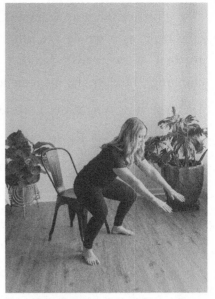

Step 4 - Bend Knees

Step 5 - Hinge Forward (Attempt to move your shoulders as far forward as possible while keeping your body weight in your midfoot.)

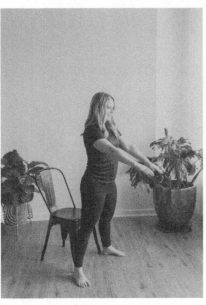

Step 6 - Stand Up

Practice these as separate exercises in addition to practicing the movement as a whole (i.e. do 10 repetitions of each movement and 10 total sit to stands). Another one of my favorite examples is stair climbing. Here are the movements you need to climb stairs effectively:

1. Shift your weight onto one leg (the leg that's on the stair).

2. Straighten that leg so you're standing on the first step.

3. Bend the opposite knee so your heel gets closer to your buttock.

4. Lift your toes/ankle.

5. Bring the knee up toward the ceiling.

6. Place the foot on the step.

7. Shift your body weight forward onto the front leg.

8. Repeat on the other side.

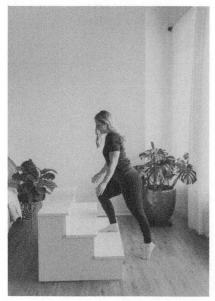 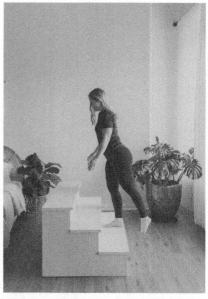

Step 1 - Shift Weight Forward **Step 2 - Step Up/Straighten Your Leg**

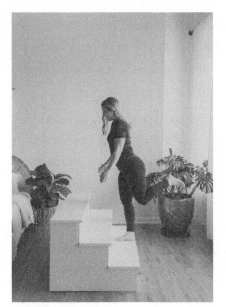

Step 3 - Bend Knee

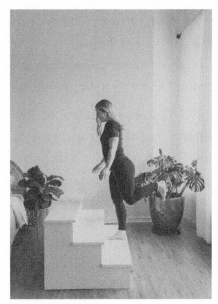

Step 4 - Lift Toes

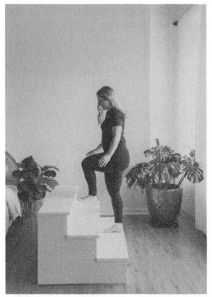

Step 5 - Bring Knee Forward

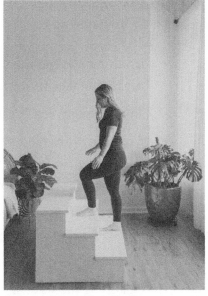

Step 6 - Place Foot Down

Note: If you're starting with both feet on the floor, you'll follow the same steps, but skip step No. 2. Similar to the previous functions, you'd use these seven steps as individual exercises. As always, use a railing and/or a mobility aid to prioritize your safety.

You are in control of your exercise routine. If you have enough energy and time to incorporate all seven walking exercises into your routine, go for it! But if that's too much, just add one or two. Performing one or two exercises consistently (i.e. five days per week) will get you to your goal faster than performing seven exercises two days per week because you don't have the time or energy to do them frequently. When selecting one or two exercises, choose the hardest ones for you to complete, since that identifies where most of your weakness lives!

One question you may be thinking is "How many repetitions should I do? How many sets should I do? How many minutes should I exercise?" In this case, refer to the information you learned in Chapter 3 on neuroplasticity. For all exercises, please implement the neuroplasticity guidelines:

- Do as many repetitions as you can with good quality. If you need a number to strive for, shoot for 30.

- Take as many rest breaks as you need.

- Exercising throughout the day is just as effective as exercising all at once, so if you prefer to exercise in small chunks of time, or don't have a full 30 minutes to exercise, split it up!

- MS research shows five to six days of exercise per week is best. Other research suggests 150 minutes per week.

- Aim to exercise for at least 30 minutes, five days a week.

- Quality is the most important factor.

- If it's impossible to have good quality, do your best with less movement instead of skipping it altogether. For example, do a marching exercise, but lift your leg up enough to where your knee doesn't fall to the outside.

- If you have no movement, it's still beneficial to do the exercise in an attempt to find a neural pathway that will eventually strengthen the muscle.

How to Improve Movement in Your Day-To-Day Life

Okay, so now you know the basics to break down your goals and turn them into functional exercises. The next step is to *implement* these movements throughout the day. If you miss this step, I can almost guarantee that you might get stronger, but your function, or activity, won't feel any easier.

Let's stick with the example of improving walking quality. Becoming aware of your current walking habits is the first step. Are you swinging (circumducting) your leg to the side to advance it forward? Are you dropping your foot or scuffing your toes? Are you not bending your knee enough? Becoming aware of the specifics can make it easier to focus on one area to prioritize.

Let's run with the idea that you have hip circumduction when walking, meaning you're swinging your leg out to the side when taking a step forward. The reason this happens can be due to weakness in bending your knee, weakness in your hip flexors, weakness in your ankle, and poor balance. Not to mention other factors like fatigue, pain, or lack of sensation. There are lots of strengthening exercises we can do to work on hip circumduction, including the ones you've learned from this chapter and previous chapters, but we also need to be aware of when we are circumducting our hips.

- Is it with every step?
- Is it just in the mornings?

- Is it just in the evenings?

- Is it only when you're fatigued?

Our brain wants to keep doing the things we repeat (ahem: neuroplasticity). Keep in mind, every time you circumduct your hip while walking, you're communicating with your brain to reinforce the leg swing. Regardless of strengthening exercises, your brain doesn't understand how to utilize your new strength.

As soon as you notice your leg swinging/circumducting, pause, remember what good quality should look and feel like, and do your best to step forward with good form. This can be challenging since the reason you're circumducting could be due to weak muscles, but this strategy is a powerful way to improve walking form and communication with your brain on how you want to move.

- Yes, it's going to slow you down.

- Yes, it's going to be hard.

- No, you don't need to have good form with every step.

So, if you notice your leg swinging while walking to the bathroom and you cannot hold it, don't worry about implementing good form at that moment. Do what you must to get to the bathroom safely. You can pick and choose the times to implement good form, but aim for at least 50 percent of the time. Think about it this way: Let's say you consistently exercise for up to one hour per day. On average, we're awake for about 16 hours, meaning that for one hour of good form, you have 15 hours of poor form. Quite frankly, strengthening with good form for one hour won't make much of a difference when it comes to function and activities. It's important to start implementing good quality and form into your day, even if it's just a few repetitions here and there.

"Exaggerated walking" is a powerful exercise because it tells the brain exactly how much effort to put into each movement. If you're doing this exercise correctly, you should feel silly when walking.

My favorite way to implement the strengthening exercises to improve walking is to practice "exaggerated walking." If you're doing this right, you should feel silly. This is a powerful exercise because it tells the brain exactly how much effort to put into each movement. You'll fatigue quickly with this exercise since it requires a lot of strength, balance, coordination, and concentration. Do this for a few steps several times a day. As you get stronger, add more steps and then add some more.

Another great example of implementing new strategies into day-to-day life is entering and exiting a car. I encourage you to use your hip flexor strength to lift your leg into and out of the car, instead of using your hands or arms to help lift your leg, if possible. If you don't practice this implementation, you might discover that your hip flexor strength has improved from your exercises, but they aren't working properly. So, this function hasn't become easier for you.

KEY TAKEAWAYS

1 The steps outlined in this chapter are helpful if you're starting from zero or you've been exercising for a few months or years.

2 Choose one or two activities in your day-to-day life that you want to be easier.

3 Create functional exercises out of the movements the activity requires.

4 Implement exercises and proper movement into your day.

5. If you need help figuring out which exercises you should prioritize, work with an MS-specialized physical therapist.

6. Have hope!

RESOURCES

- To get a pdf & video demonstration of each exercise shown in this book, head to:
  https://www.doctorgretchenhawley.com/bookpdf

- The MSing Link podcast episode No. 9, "Improve Your Movement Through Functional Exercise"

- Check out functional exercises on my YouTube page.

Visit: https://www.youtube.com/c/DoctorGretchenHawley

CHAPTER 6

Modify Your Exercises to Work for You

You know the difference between functional and traditional exercises, but maybe you're a bit stumped, especially if you lack the strength to practice in a functional position. And, where do you work out if you don't have a gym membership or lack the space at home? Have no fear, there's always a way to exercise functionally, regardless of your current level of strength, balance, flexibility, or energy level.

First, let's talk about exercise positions, then locations within the home. The two most common exercise positions for improving walking strength and endurance, standing endurance, reducing foot drop, climbing stairs, and standing up and sitting down without plopping down, are sitting and standing. In those movements, you're either in a sitting or standing position, so the most functional exercise position includes those two.

If fatigue, poor balance, pain, or the inability to get out of bed or off the couch are an issue, a backup option is crucial. Otherwise, you won't exercise at all if it's difficult or impossible to start in the functional position.

Position Options for Exercising

1. **Standing:** There are lots of variations. Hold on to something for balance, or not. Stand with the feet wide apart, close together, or in a staggered stance. Standing exercises are easier since the hips are extended, but they can also be challenging since it requires balance and good posture. Do your best to make sure your knees are not locked or hyperextended, if possible, to prevent knee pain and further muscle weakness in your thigh muscles.

2. **Sitting:** Sit upright for a more challenging position since the hips are more flexed, or recline backward for an easier version since the hips are more extended. It's important to activate the abdominal muscles when sitting upright or reclined, otherwise, the back muscles may start to overcompensate, which can cause lower back discomfort or pain.

3. **Lying on your back (supine):** Lie on your back on the bed, couch, treatment table, bench, or the ground. Make sure to choose a surface that you can safely and comfortably stand up from. Your legs can be straight or you can place a pillow under your knees, if that's more comfortable for your back. This position can be great for stretching, but challenging for strengthening since most exercises in this position require you to lift a body part (i.e. leg) up against gravity.

4. **Lying on your back with knees bent (hook lying):** Same as above, but the knees are bent and facing the ceiling with the

feet firmly planted on the surface (the bed, couch or floor). This position is often more comfortable than supine. However, it can be more challenging to stabilize the hips, making your legs feel more wobbly.

5. **Lying on your side (side lying):** Typically, it's easiest to lie on your strongest side. For example, if your right leg is stronger than the left, practice the side-lying exercises on your right side to make the movements a little bit easier. Then, on the next set, turn over to the left side. This position takes gravity out of the situation, making the exercise less challenging.

6. **Lying on your stomach (prone):** There are some variations to this position, depending on how it feels for your body. One option is to lie fully flat with your chest, hips, knees, and toes all touching the surface. You can choose how you want to rest your head. This position can cause discomfort for anyone with hip flexor tightness, so place a pillow underneath the hips to make this position more comfortable.

7. **On your hands and knees (quadruped):** This is the least common exercise position, since it can be challenging to get into. But this position is where you'll be when you're getting up from the floor, so it's a functional position.

In the photos below, I demonstrate one exercise in each of these positions. The exercise I'm demonstrating is one of my all-time favorites because it helps with so many functions including walking, climbing stairs, getting up from the ground, getting into and out of a car, bed, or shower. The exercise is marching. Keep in mind that each position strengthens the hip flexor muscles.

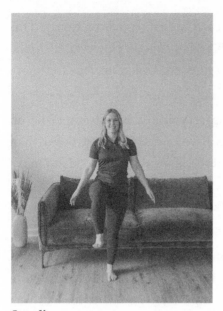

Standing

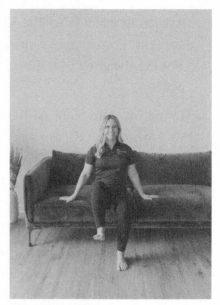

Sitting Upright

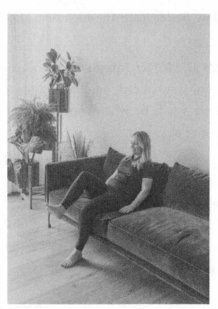

Sitting Reclined

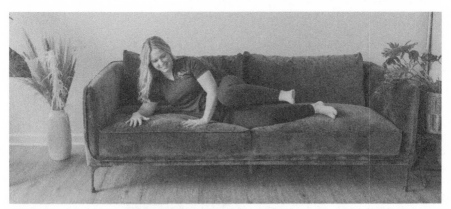

Sidelying - Bring one or both knees up

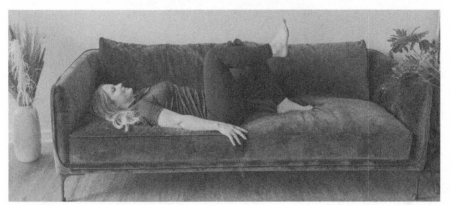

Hooklying

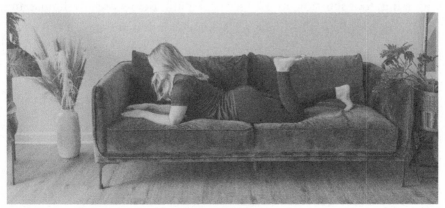

Prone - Push your knee down into the couch

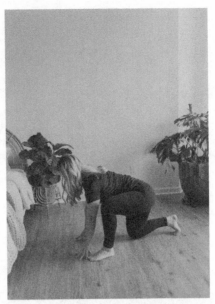

Quadruped - Start with both knees on the ground, then bring one knee forward and place your foot on the ground, then return to the start position.

Below, you'll find another example of how to perform an exercise in various positions. This time, "hamstring curls" a.k.a.: bending your knee to strengthen your hamstrings. Stronger hamstrings equal improved walking, stair climbing, and posture with reduced hip swinging, foot scuffing, and lower back pain. Below are five hamstring curl positions. Pick which one feels doable for you any day of the week.

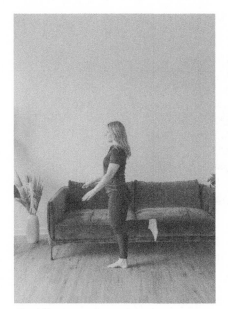

Standing

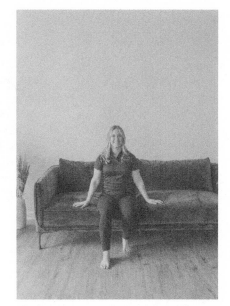

Sitting

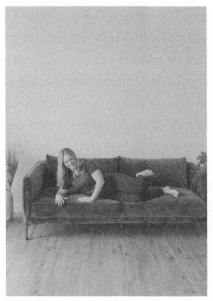

Sidelying

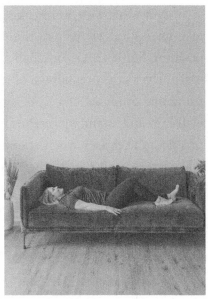

Supine

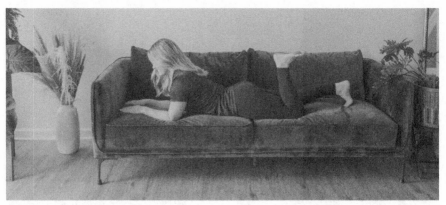

Prone

As you can see, there are pros and cons to every position. Every exercise requires different muscles, meaning some positions will be easier for some and harder for others. Remember that these are all options. You do not need to perform every exercise in every position. Choose which position feels best to you.

Now that you know the positions, go ahead and pick one to take for a spin. My rule of thumb is to start with the most functional position, but if that's too challenging, choose a different option that's easier. Here's the breakdown of how I'd prioritize the exercise positions using one of my MSing Link members who is working on improving walking and standing endurance, as an example. We'd begin by practicing exercises when standing since we're in a standing position when we're walking. If that's too challenging, she can practice the same exercise sitting upright or reclined. If that's still too hard, the next option is to practice the same exercise when hook-lying. If that's too difficult, she'll attempt the exercise side-lying. Once she finds a position that is doable, this will become part of her home routine.

There's a lot of trial and error involved but our goal is to find a position where the exercise can be successfully performed for several repetitions (up to 15 good-quality repetitions with or without rest breaks). There's no right or wrong. Once you're stronger in the less functional position, pick another position, and so on until you're practicing in the most functional position!

Here's How You'll Know if It's Time to Exercise in a Different Position:

1. If the movement you're aiming for isn't happening. For example, if you try to lift your leg, but there is very little or no movement.

2. If there is pain or increased discomfort with the exercise.

3. If it's difficult or impossible to get into the functional position.

4. If there's poor quality with the exercise. For example, if you lift your leg and your knee falls outward causing your ankle to angle inward toward your opposite leg. For this movement, good quality doesn't include angling. The knee comes straight up toward the ceiling and the ankle stays in alignment with the knee.

I often recommend starting with the easiest position. When the exercise is easier, you can knock out good quality repetitions, leading to more opportunities for your brain to strengthen or find new neural pathways, which is the whole point.

Location, Location, Location

When thinking about functional exercises, it's also important to consider functional locations. For example, if the goal is to climb the stairs with ease—without using your arms to pull yourself up—then one of the most functional places to perform this movement is the stairs in your house. Can you hit the gym? Yes. But sometimes those locations come with their own set of difficulties, due to the energy and time commitment required to leave the house, exercise, and return home. Let's talk about the locations in your home.

> If your goal is to climb the stairs with ease—without using your arms to pull yourself up—then one of the most functional places to perform this movement is the stairs in your house.

There are two ways to determine your at-home exercise location. The first is to think of the most functional spot. Remember your goals and identify which rooms align with those goals. For example:

- Want to climb stairs with ease? Exercise on your stairs.

- Want to stand up off your couch with ease? Exercise on your couch.

- Want to sit down without plopping on the toilet? Exercise on the toilet.

- Want to grab your laundry without losing your balance? Exercise at your washer or dryer.

- Want to squat down low enough to pick up the dog's food dish? Exercise in the kitchen.

- Want to put on your pants or socks without losing balance? Exercise in your bedroom.

Each of the locations above come with variations. Let's use the stairs as our example. There are exercises you can do when facing the stairs or facing sideways. When exercising on the couch, the options are to exercise lying down supine, hook lying, lying on your side, sitting unsupported, or sitting supported by the back of the couch. There are lots of choices once you get to the location. My favorite exercise locations are the couch, bed, toilet (stand up and sit down multiple times), near the kitchen or bathroom sink, and at the kitchen or dining room table. That said, I'm always up for getting creative. If I have a client who desires to improve balance while reaching for a sweater in their closet, then they practice balance and weight-shifting exercises in the closet! If a client has difficulty getting out of bed, then they'll practice exercises in their bed.

The trick is to make the exercise easier at first in order to find sustainable success. For example, if the goal is to stand up from the couch with better strength and balance (not plopping down), then practicing standing up from the couch might be too challenging—at first. Put an extra cushion on the couch, so that it's higher than the normal cushion. Next, practice standing up and sitting down from the higher surface until your strength improves. Then, remove the extra cushion and practice from a lower height.

The other type of location to exercise is wherever it's easiest for you. After a long day at work, you might not feel like finding a functional at-home exercise location. Guess what? You don't have to. Perform the exercises at the dining room table. Or do all of your standing exercises at the kitchen sink. Any immovable surface (i.e. no wheels) is a good place for seated exercises. Any surface with a safety net (in case you lose your balance) is a safe place to perform standing exercises. Avoid wet or damp surfaces since that could cause a fall. If you can multitask, watch TV while exercising.

What To Do if You're Having a Bad Day

A bad day looks different for each person with MS, and will vary in intensity, symptoms, and duration. That's why it's important to have a strategy in place on those bad days, which may include:

- little to no energy
- increased pain
- worsened sensory symptoms (numbness, tingling, etc.)
- increased weakness
- poor balance
- being mentally drained

I Have Three Strategies for Bad Days:

1. **Rest, guilt-free:** The body NEEDS rest. Muscles grow during rest days. Does your body need more rest than most? Maybe! But that's not a reason to neglect it. If your body craves rest, give it rest. This may mean pausing your exercise routine for one day or several days in a row. When you're resting, adopt the mindset that you're doing something good for your body. Don't feel guilty. Guilt does nothing but drain your energy. Did you ever notice how guilty rest isn't as peaceful as guilt-free rest? Try your best not to judge yourself. You deserve to rest. If you need rest but know your body feels better with some movement, move on to strategy No. 2.

2. **All movement counts:** That's right, walking around the house, fetching the mail, showering, getting dressed, and cooking counts! With all of these activities, muscles are activating and engaged.

One of my MSing Link members, Christine, felt guilty about skipping exercises several days in a row. When I asked why she'd skipped them, she said: "My daughter has been very sick. She's staying in her room upstairs to avoid infecting the rest of our family. I've been taking care of her bringing her soup, Kleenex, and anything else she needs."

Then, I asked about the number of stairs from the first floor to the second floor. There were two flights with about 20 or so steps, which Christine climbed several times a day to care for her daughter.

This meant Christine climbed those steps about five times per day, totalling 80 to 100 steps per day. And she walked around her home cooking, doing laundry, and other daily chores. I explained to Christine that all of this movement counted as exercise, even though it wasn't part of her normal routine. "That explains why I'm so tired and sore," she replied. "I feel better knowing these movements count as exercise!"

3. **Modify the exercise:** First and foremost, choose the easiest exercise. This way you'll perform it successfully with good form. If you need to modify the easiest exercise (or any exercise for that matter) choose a different/easier position or location. For example, choose a higher surface to practice standing up. Or practice leg kicks right from the edge of your bed or couch. Next, perform fewer reps (i.e. five repetitions instead of 20 to 30), move faster (faster is easier than slower), hold for less time (i.e. hold the exercise for one second instead of three), and take more rest breaks. You can implement all of these strategies or just a few. It's up to you and how much you want to push yourself.

Most importantly, listen to your body.

> Not sure if you're performing each exercise correctly because you don't see any movement? Place one or two fingers on the muscle that should be activated. Then, perform the movement and check to see if you can feel anything under your fingertips.

For example, perform the seated marching exercise while you're touching your hip flexors. As you attempt to lift your leg into a march, notice any sensation of muscle tightening under your fingers. If you don't feel anything, relax, move your fingers to a different spot, and try the exercise again. Often, when you don't have enough strength to lift your leg, your muscles may still be working. This is a sign that the neural pathways are there and activating, but aren't strong enough (yet) to lift the leg. Stay at it, rinse and repeat. Consider yourself successful based on the effort applied to each repetition.

KEY TAKEAWAYS

1. You can exercise in seven main positions, including: standing, sitting upright or reclined, supine, hook lying, side lying, quadruped, and prone.

2. When choosing an exercise position or location, start with a goal. Choose the most functional position and location, if possible. Feel free to exercise in any room of your house.

3. On bad days, participate in guilt-free rest; get any form of movement or modify your exercise routine. Listen to your body.

4. Have hope! Because your mind and movement depend on it.

RESOURCES

- To get a pdf & video demonstration of each exercise shown in this book, head to:
  https://www.doctorgretchenhawley.com/bookpdf

- The MSing Link podcast episode No. 93, "Exercise Positions & Locations"

CHAPTER 7

Measure Your Progress at Home

W hen you go to a physical therapy clinic, there are specific tests to evaluate strength, flexibility, balance, etc. Some of these tests are also used at your neurology clinic as a baseline and recurring measurement to track progress. Examples of these tests include:

Manual muscle testing: This is used to measure strength in specific muscle groups, including hip flexors and extensors, hip rotators, knee flexors and extensors, ankle flexors, and many more. It's graded on a scale from 0 to 5 with 0 indicating no strength and 5 indicating full strength.

Balance: These tests are used to measure balance in different positions, which gives your physical therapist an idea of what your balance might be like in real-life situations. During the tests, you'll stand with your feet apart, together, in a staggered stance, and with a tandem stance. Additionally, your seated balance may be tested to check your core strength. Generally speaking, if you can maintain balance in a position for 20 seconds, you've passed the test, indicating it may not be a priority for your therapy sessions.

Muscle tightness/spasticity: As you may suspect, this is used to measure the tightness of your muscles. Tight muscles make moving and walking more challenging because it prevents full muscle use. Each muscle can be tested individually to get an accurate assessment of the degree of tightness. This is often graded using the Modified Ashworth Scale which indicates the level of spasticity. The scale is as follows:

- Grade 0: No increase in tone/tightness.

- Grade 1: Slight increase in tone; the physical therapist might be able to move your limb freely but then feel a "catch" or resistance at the end of the motion.

- Grade 1+: Slight increase in tone, but the catch or resistance is felt throughout half of the range of motion, not just at the end.

- Grade 2: The physical therapist is still able to move your limb throughout the whole motion, but there is increased tone throughout the entire range of motion.

- Grade 3: Considerable increase in tone; the physical therapist will likely struggle to move your limb throughout half of your range of motion.

- Grade 4: Rigid; the PT will likely not be able to move the limb at all.

This test can be very subjective. Your score may vary slightly from one physical therapist to another. However, it's the only test at this time designed to accurately measure spasticity.

Range of motion: This is used to measure joint mobility. One reason walking and other movements may be challenging is due to weak or tight muscles, but another is lack of mobility can be found in the joint. Range of motion may be limited due to an injury, swelling, arthritis, increased cartilage build-up, joint misalignment, or pain. Typically, this test is measured in degrees. For example, your knee bends 135 degrees.

Coordination: Coordination plays a huge role in maintaining balance and the smoothness of your gait. Impaired coordination impacts strength, speed, and precision of lower limb movement resulting in "walking like you're drunk" or poor foot placement when walking. Coordination can be measured using your upper or lower body. When assessing via the upper body, you may be asked to touch your finger to your nose then reach forward to touch the physical therapist's finger; you'll repeat this movement several times. When assessing via the lower body, you may be asked to tap your foot or place your heel to your shin repeatedly. These are just a few of the many coordination tests available.

Functional outcome tests/measures: These are either subjective (self-evaluated) or objective (measurable) tests that are used to quantify improvement in function, such as walking speed, standing up, sitting down, mobility from a seated position, balance while walking, and leg strength. The most common functional outcome test you've likely performed at your neurologist's office or physical therapy clinic is the Timed 25-Foot Walk Test. Theoretically, the more consistent you are with your exercises, the more likely you'll see improvement in these tests over time. In the next few pages, I'll outline functional outcome tests that, according to Dr. Gabriel Pardo from Oklahoma Medical Research Foundation 2021 findings in his study "Outcome Measures Assisting Treatment Optimization in Multiple Sclerosis" are the most effective tests to accurately measure progress for people with MS.

Other areas where the physical therapist may assess on evaluation day and during re-evaluation visits are vision, sensation, swelling/blood flow, aerobic endurance, and others. All of these tests are used to track progress and show insurance companies how you're doing with physical therapy and if it's "working" or not. Unfortunately, one of the insurance company's main goals is to get you out of PT as quickly as possible, even though you have a progressive disease. Often, if you're improving, they may believe you've improved enough. Or, if you're not improving, they think you aren't going to improve. In both cases, and far too often, their suggestion is to discharge you from PT. It's a tricky game that isn't fair to those with chronic illnesses. But this isn't necessarily the end. Often, the physical therapist can appeal the denial by offering more detailed information and pleading your case. This can result in approval of more PT sessions.

At-Home Tests to Measure Progress

A disappointing aspect of our healthcare system is that once a patient is discharged from physical therapy, it can be harder to track their progress; and it's difficult for them to stay consistent with their exercises. This sometimes leads to losing months or years of progress. Your neurologist may measure some of these tests, but that usually happens only once or twice a year.

Are you ready for the good news? There is a way to modify functional outcome measures, allowing the patient to perform them at home.

> All of my clients who track their progress with at-home tests stay more consistent with their exercises, feel more motivated, and see improvements in their strength and mobility.

You can also track these tests while you're actively in physical therapy or start them when you're discharged from PT. I'll be the first to admit there are more inconsistent variables with at-home testing, which means the results might not be as accurate as those found in a clinical setting. However, it's a great workaround for those motivated by tracking and seeing a difference in their scores.

Let's get to the good stuff. Here are the most effective functional outcome measures for people with MS combined with my twist on how you can apply them at home. According to Dr. Pardo's research, these tests are the most likely to pick up on subtle differences, indicating improvements, maintenance, or regression.

Subjective Functional Outcome Measures for MS (Self-Reported)

1. **Modified Fatigue Impact Scale (MFIS):** This 21-item questionnaire assesses how fatigue influences physical, cognitive, and psychosocial functioning. Each item asks how fatigue has impacted your life in specific situations within the last four weeks. You'll rate the severity of fatigue on a scale of 0-4. For example: 0 indicates no impact, while four indicates you were almost always impacted. The total MFIS score will range from 0 to 84. The higher the score, the higher the impact. The goal, of course, is to exercise consistently and implement other symptom management strategies such as energy conservation to lower the score. Energy conservation techniques are ways to conserve your energy, such as sitting while cooking instead of standing, letting your dishes air dry instead of drying them yourself, or taking seated breaks during a chore or task.

2. **Multiple Sclerosis Walking Scale-12 (MSWS-12):** This 12-item questionnaire assesses walking ability. Each item asks how MS has affected your walking in specific situations within the last two weeks. The scoring provides options 1 through 5 for each item; with 1 indicating no effect and 5 indicating an extreme effect. The total MSWS-12 score can range from 12 to 60. Higher scores

indicate a greater impact on walking than lower scores. Again, if you are consistent with your exercise routine, your walking should improve and your score should drop.

Objective Functional Outcome Measures for MS

1. **Timed 25-foot walk test:** This walking test to assess speed is the most common functional outcome measure you've likely performed annually at the neurologist's office and frequently at the physical therapist's clinic. At the clinic, patients are timed as they walk 25 feet from one marked point to another.

   To do this test at home, grab a stopwatch and determine two immovable points that are about 25 feet apart, with a clear pathway. Maybe it's one end of the hallway to the other or one doorway to another doorway. If you have one, grab the measuring tape to check the distance. It's okay to modify this test with two landmarks that are less than or greater than the classic 25 feet. Make note of the landmarks so you can replicate the test each time you perform it. Set the time on the stopwatch then walk as quickly as you can while maintaining safety. My clients perform this test three times, then take the average score.

2. **Timed Up & Go (TUG):** This test attempts to quantify functional mobility. To do this test at home, you'll need a cleared walkway between a sturdy chair (i.e. couch, sofa, or dining room chair pushed up against a wall) and an immovable object (kitchen table, doorway, or window), and a timer. Ask a friend or family member to work the timer so you focus on taking the test. The distance between the chair and the immovable object should be about three meters, but since this is at your home it doesn't need to be exact. Start in a seated position in the chair. Next, time how long it takes you to stand up, walk to your immovable object, turn around, walk back to the chair, turn around and sit down. (Tip: If needed, use the chair's armrests to push off and help you stand up and sit down

safely. Also, if you normally use a walking aid, use it during this test.)

3. **Two or Six-Minute Walk Test:** This test measures self-paced walking ability and functional capacity. The original test required the patient to walk for six minutes, but the modified version is widely used since, at two-minutes long, it's much shorter. To perform this test at home, you'll need a stopwatch and mobility aid, if you use one. This test is fairly simple, but not easy. To complete the test, walk for two minutes straight in an obstacle-free pathway. As with the other tests, it's best to start in the same spot and take the same path each time you perform this test. Make sure you choose an immovable starting point, such as a doorway, window, or wall. Your pathway could be a long hallway, laps around the kitchen, or laps around the perimeter of several rooms. As long as you walk the same path each time, it doesn't matter what path you take.

There are two ways to track the results. The first option is to measure the distance walked in two minutes. This is easiest if you stay on a straight path on a long hallway. If you know the distance of the hallway, multiply that metric by the number of times you walked the corridor. The second option is to track the number of laps walked around the different rooms. Maybe you walked the hallway 10 times. Or maybe you walked the perimeter of the living room and kitchen five times.

There are plenty of other functional outcome measures to perform such as the Five Times Sit to Stand Test, Dynamic Gait Index (DGI), BERG Balance Scale, and the Functional Gait Assessment (FGA) to name a few. These tests garner the biggest bang for your buck when it comes to effective MS analysis. Pick and choose which tests to perform or do them on different days to avoid fatigue. The goal is to make these tests as accurate and reproducible as possible, especially since

MS symptoms vary so much from day to day. Tracking all measures possible and collecting accurate data is vitally important.

First, choose the time of day to perform these tests. For example, if the first time you perform the TUG and the 25-foot walk test is at 10 a.m. on a fatigue- and symptom-free day, don't repeat it four weeks later at 5 p.m. when you're extra fatigued. I get it, this may be challenging since MS varies from day to day, but do your best. Don't worry about perfection.

Second, recreate the test using the same objects. If anything changes, write it down in your notes. This helps because if your numbers vary from previous recordings, the new objects could be the culprit.

Third, mobility aids are always welcome. Do your best to maintain safety during all of these tests. Often, this means using a mobility aid or other devices, like an AFO, Bioness, or Dictus Band. In your notes, record which mobility aids and devices were used for each test. You can take it one step further and write down how much you depended on the mobility aid (i.e. 50 percent).

Your walking quality in each walking-based test is important. I'd even say it's more important than the time you score. Often, when your legs get stronger, your walking will slow down—initially. Your TUG and/or timed 25-foot walk test may show a slower time, but there was a reduced number of foot scuffs and zero missteps. Now that's an improvement! While the time of each test is important, the quality is equally important. Make notes about foot scuffs, how much you're bending your knee, if your hip is swinging around (circumducting) and if you're hinging forward.

Want to start tracking these tests? Download The MSing Link app along with the video-based instructions for each test. This may be an unpopular opinion, but take some of these subjective tests, like the manual muscle testing and MRI, with a grain of salt. Keep in mind:

How you're feeling is more important than what some of these tests reveal. One of my clients, Mary, had been working on her MSing Link exercises consistently. She felt stronger, her walking improved, and she maneuvered around the house with better balance. However, Mary was shocked and confused when the neurologist said her legs were testing weaker than her previous visit. Sadly, Mary got discouraged and lost the motivation to exercise. After she explained the situation, I said: "Mary, do you FEEL weaker?"

She replied, "No."

"Have you noticed weakness when going about your day-to-day life?" I asked.

Again, she replied, "No."

Then, I explained a simple truth to Mary. While the manual muscle testing showed weakness, if it didn't impact her day-to-day life, she shouldn't let the test results get her down. Why? Because she had proof. Consistent exercise had helped her daily movements.

KEY TAKEAWAYS

1. The neurologist's office and physical therapy clinic have many tests to track progress, maintenance, and/or regression of strength and function. And there are ways to modify these tests to do them at home.

2. Subjective functional outcome measures are self-reported tests based on how you feel about fatigue, walking quality, and other symptoms. According to research, the most effective subjective tests for MS are the Modified Fatigue Impact Scale (MFIS) and the Multiple Sclerosis Walking Scale-12 (MSWS-12).

3. Objective functional outcome measures are based on measurable data to quantify movement, strength, etc. According to research, the most effective objective tests are the 25-foot walk test, timed

up and go (TUG), two-minute walk test, and the five times sit to stand test.

4 Stay safe when performing these tests at home. Use mobility aids, arm rests, whatever is necessary to avoid injury. Ask a friend or family member to time your objective tests. Focus on how you feel and your walking quality, not the test itself. This is often a better indicator of progress.

5 Have hope! Be consistent. Even if that means exercising two to three days per week. You've got this!

RESOURCES

- The MSing Link podcast episode No. 111, - "How to Measure Progress At Home"
- Download The MSing Link app for iOS or Android and view demonstrations in the "tracking" section

CHAPTER 8

Relapse or Pseudo-Relapse?
That is The Question

An MS relapse can be extremely scary and nerve-wracking (no pun intended). There are two main types of relapses: a true relapse and a pseudo relapse. You're about to learn why they happen and a plan of attack, if and when you experience a relapse.

A true multiple sclerosis relapse, also known as an attack, flare, or exacerbation, is when any new symptom(s) arises. Or, an old symptom that's been gone for at least a month returns, accompanied by new plaque formations seen on an MRI. The cause? Neuro-inflammation in your brain, spinal cord, or optic nerves. When inflammation is present, parts of your neural pathways get blocked resulting in miscommunication between your brain and your muscles. This can lead to various symptoms such as weakness in a different muscle, vision changes, sensory changes, slurred speech, memory changes, imbalance, etc. The severity can be very mild or severe enough that it interferes with your day-to-day life. The symptoms typically last longer than 24 hours and do not go away unless treated by a neurologist.

A pseudo-relapse is the temporary worsening of one or multiple symptoms you've previously experienced. There is no new demyelination or damage to the brain, spinal cord, or optic nerves. Rather, it's caused by triggers such as fever, physical or mental stress, trauma, depression, heat or cold intolerance, change in core temperature, or any type of infection. This trigger can temporarily activate an old lesion. Symptoms usually dissipate within 24 hours, but sometimes they last for 48 hours.

How to Differentiate Between a True Relapse and a Pseudo-Relapse

If your answer is yes to the questions below, you're experiencing a pseudo-relapse. If your answer is no, you're experiencing a true relapse.

1. Is this a symptom you've felt before?

2. Did the symptom last less than 48 hours?

3. Are you experiencing any triggers that may be causing worsened symptoms like heat intolerance, stress, or an infection? If you're not sure, get tested for a UTI or another infection that may be starting.

Whether it's a true relapse or a pseudo-relapse it's important to contact your neurologist and healthcare team as soon as you experience new or worsening symptoms lasting more than 24 hours. Use the questions above as the source of information to communicate to your neurologist. Describe the new or worsening symptom, explain how long it's lasted, and detail any triggers that made the symptom worse. This will help your doctor determine if you need to be treated in the clinic or not. If your doctor recommends a visit, the physician is likely to test for a urinary tract infection (UTI), upper respiratory infection (URI), or other infections to rule out neuro-inflammation triggers. The doctor may suggest an MRI. If this is the case, don't panic! This is a standard procedure to gain more insight about what's causing the symptom. It does not necessarily mean the disease is progressing.

Treating True Relapses

Typically, for true relapses, the first line of attack is intravenous (IV) high-dose corticosteroids. These steroids are potent anti-inflammatory agents, most commonly Solumedrol, which is given via an IV for the span of five days. Another option is oral prednisone pills, also taken for five days. Occasionally, the timeline can vary based on your specific situation. While these are the most effective ways to treat relapses, they may be contraindicated for people with diabetes or gestational diabetes, ulcers, a history of gastrointestinal (GI) bleeds, or a history of psychosis with steroids. Always discuss these conditions with your neurologist and primary care physician so they can implement the best course of action for your relapse.

If treatment with steroids is unsuccessful, second-line therapies such as Acthar Gel, Intravenous Immunoglobulin (IVIG) or Total Plasma Exchange (TPE) are often considered for patients who haven't recovered from severe attacks. These may be scary or confusing words, so let's break them down:

- Acthar Gel is a hormone injected into the skin, which causes the body to make its own steroids.

- IVIG therapy is when antibodies from healthy donors are administered to you via IV.

- TPE, also known as Total Plasmapheresis, is when blood is removed from the body, filtered, and then put back into the body. This often requires five to seven exchanges every other day. It usually takes up to 14 days to complete.

Additionally, referrals to physical therapy, speech therapy, occupational therapy, and/or cognitive behavioral therapy may be recommended to maintain or improve a patient's symptoms.

Treating Pseudo-Relapses

For pseudo-relapses, the neurologist may suggest antibiotics for infections, increased rest, stress-reducing activities, and a temporary medication—such as Diazepam or Flexeril for muscle relaxation or CBD for stress reduction—in an attempt to lessen specific symptoms. Once the trigger of the pseudo-relapse is cleared, the symptoms should dissipate.

> The real doozie is that all relapses, even pseudo-relapses, may have long-lasting effects beyond the 48-hour guideline, especially if the pseudo-relapse was caused by an infection or illness. Our bodies need time to heal from an infection and it takes even longer for someone with MS.

In my experience, pseudo-relapse symptoms caused by an infection (of any kind) will plateau and stay present until the infection clears. After that, it's likely the person will return where they were, physically, before the infection.

Take MSing Link member, Ed, for example. Ed had been consistently performing his MSing Link exercises at home several times per week focusing on strengthening, balance, and endurance. After a few months, he was able to walk longer distances without a limp. He also had better balance and his foot didn't scuff the ground. Then, he got the flu and quickly lost all of the progress he'd made during our work together.

Ed drastically modified his exercises to perform the movements successfully without fatigue and he stayed as consistent as possible. He intentionally rested daily and moved his body via light exercise up to twice per week. It took four weeks for him to fully recover from the flu. Then he was ready to dial up the exercise intensity to regain the strength, balance, and energy he'd lost. After six weeks, Ed was back to his pre-flu status.

Another MSing Link member, Sarah, developed COVID which caused her to lose all progress with her exercises. She went from walking around her home with good quality to being confined to the bed for up to two weeks due to extreme weakness and fatigue. She also temporarily lost bladder control and had worsened sensitivity in her feet and hands. It took Sarah five weeks to recover from the illness before she could fully jump back into the MSing Link program. However, after six more weeks, Sarah, like Ed, was back to her pre-COVID self. This meant Sarah was able to walk at home and work without a mobility aid (with good quality), tripping less, and with increased energy.

Differentiating between a true relapse and a pseudo-relapse is important for treatment purposes and mentally knowing what to expect. New or worsening symptoms can be shocking, but increased anxiety when any symptom increases is exhausting. If you approach each worsening symptom with the mindset of determining a potential trigger, reducing that trigger, and waiting it out 24 to 48 hours, you'll (hopefully) remain calm and notice symptom relief sooner, if it's a pseudo-relapse. If not, have confidence that your doctor has various treatment methods that can help.

Each relapse and pseudo-relapse can feel different. It's important to take notes, share the information with your healthcare team if the symptoms last more than 24 hours, and take slow breaths to calm your mind and nervous system. Additionally, follow up with your healthcare provider four to six weeks after treatment if your symptoms are still present.

Disease Modifying Therapies (DMT's) attempt to prevent or lessen the likelihood of true relapses, while pseudo-relapses are prevented or lessened by monitoring day-to-day activities to stay healthy and reduce the likelihood of illness or infection, reducing stress, and maintaining a neutral core temperature. This can be managed through nutrition, complementary therapies, meditation, breathwork, etc. My current favorite stress reduction technique is coloring in a coloring book.

Exercise and Relapses: Do or Don't?

Clients and MSing Link members ask if they should exercise during a relapse. Honestly, this is not a yes or no question. The answer depends on the severity of the attack. The guidelines below are for a true relapse or a pseudo-relapse:

1. Listen to your body. If you need rest, do so without feeling guilty about it. If your symptoms are mild, continue to exercise in a way that doesn't exacerbate them. If you're able to exercise regularly, you may need to modify some or all of the exercises.

2. If you can't exercise but don't need to rest, participate in any form of movement. This can mean walking around the house; moving your upper body when sitting on a couch or in bed; standing up and sitting down several times. Movement counts as exercise.

3. The more you move and exercise during a relapse, the more likely you'll recover faster once the relapse clears - even if the exercise is less strenuous than what you're used to doing.

If the relapse was severe and you lost a lot of strength, balance, mobility, etc., implement the exercise modifications you learned earlier in this book. To recap, **change the location of your exercise.** You have permission to exercise from bed or your couch. **Change your**

physical position. Lie down or sit the whole time if you'd like. **Move at a speed that makes it easier. Do fewer repetitions. Take more rest breaks. Do fewer exercises.** Start with just one or two exercises for a few days that week. Once you're ready, add a third exercise. Once you've added three or four exercises, focus on doing them more days throughout the week. Eventually, build up to about five to six exercises for five to six days per week, if your body can tolerate that. This may take months to achieve after a relapse. That's okay. Go slow and steady. Trust the process.

KEY TAKEAWAYS

1. A true relapse is a new symptom lasting more than 48 hours, accompanied by new changes on an MRI. True relapses are caused by the disease process of MS and are often treated with high-dose corticosteroids followed by second-line therapies, such as IVIG, TPE or Acthar Gel.

2. A pseudo-relapse is a temporary worsening of a current symptom that usually lessens or fully disappears after 24 to 48 hours. It's caused by a trigger, often a fever or infection, stress, trauma, etc. Treatment includes managing the infection or fever and lowering stress, etc.

3. Contact your neurologist and healthcare team if new or worsening symptoms last more than 24 hours.

4. Exercising is safe during a relapse, but listen to your body and don't push yourself. If possible, modify your exercise routine so you're able to maintain as much strength as you can until you're fully healed and ready to bump up your routine.

5. Have hope! Relapses happen, but the treatments are effective; and the likelihood of getting back to where you were before the relapse is high. You've got this!

RESOURCES

- The MSing Link podcast episode No. 117, "Relapse vs. Pseudo-Relapse"

CHAPTER 9

Mobility Aids: Good or Evil?

There's a stigma around using a mobility aid, but before we go there, let's discuss the two types of mobility training: neuro recovery and compensation. The exercises and strategies you've learned thus far taught you neuro-recovery training. The goal with neuro recovery is to perform exercises that'll help muscles get stronger (over time) through neuroplasticity. Compensation training focuses on providing alternate exercises, tools, and aids that allow you to perform all of your day-to-day activities.

> While some gain strength and mobility through neuroplasticity and neuro recovery training within a few weeks or months, others can take upward of one to two years. So, it can be helpful to implement compensation training at the same time.

This combination allows you to focus on getting stronger, while also participating in your daily activities and increasing mobility by using a tool or an aid.

- An example of a neuro-recovery-based exercise for getting into bed or a car is marching. This exercise strengthens the hip flexors, which are needed to lift your leg up and into the car.

- An example of a compensation strategy for improving the same activity is to use your arms to lift your leg into a bed or car.

- An example of a compensation tool to improve the ease of getting into a bed or a car is to use a leg lifter. This tool looks like a dog leash, but has metal on the inside which makes it more rigid. There is a loop at the bottom and at the top to hook your foot around one end and your hands around the other. From there, use your arm and hand strength to lift your leg up and into the car.

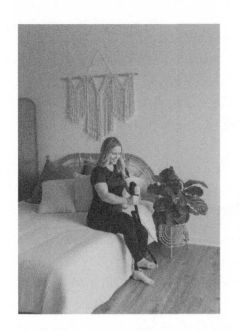
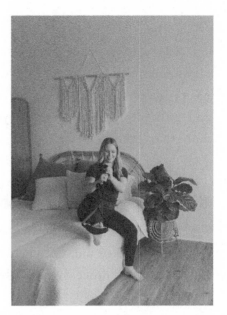
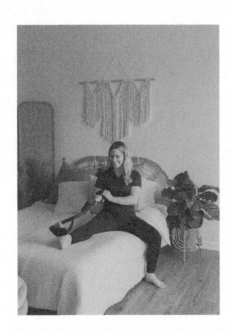

All of the compensation tools and aids mentioned in this chapter can help you stay independent and functional throughout your day. Using them does not mean you're aging or giving up or that your MS has progressed. It simply means you're taking charge of your mobility and utilizing tools to improve your strength, balance, and walking more than exercise alone.

When to Consider Using a Mobility Aid or Helpful Tool

Knowing when to start using a mobility aid, swapping one for a different mobility aid, or when to use a helpful tool can be tricky. Luckily, some telltale signs will indicate when it's time to make a change.

If you're tripping more than usual: This indicates worsening balance, more weakness, increased fatigue, and/or poor coordination, which can be improved through exercises in addition to a mobility aid.

If you're falling more often: Let me clarify something. A "fall" is anytime you end up on the floor, even if it was slow, controlled, and you didn't get hurt. The truth is, most falls are controlled. Mobility aids can make falls less likely to happen.

If you're isolating yourself: Fatigue is one of the most common causes of isolation. Let's be honest, getting dressed, leaving the house, and meeting up with friends or family, then coming home can be physically and mentally draining. Mobility aids reduce fatigue and improve mobility, allowing you to enjoy more time with friends and family.

If you're sedentary: Fatigue and difficulty with movement can lead to a sedentary lifestyle. Of course, exercises can improve your strength and mobility, but that takes time. Mobility aids can help improve your mobility right away, leading to a less sedentary life. Even if that means you're walking around your home more frequently.

If you're getting weaker: If you're noticing any undesired movements such as knee buckling/giving way, knee hyperextension, drop foot, imbalance, walking like you're drunk, or any unintended movement, it's a sign that weakness is influencing your mobility. Mobility aids can also improve your strength.

Which Mobility Aid Should You Try?

Fortunately, there are several types of mobility aids, ranging from minimal to maximum support. The mobility aid should align with how much support is needed to stay safe while walking. Your physical therapist can help you determine which one(s) are the most beneficial for you. Below are some of the most common mobility aids that I suggest to my clients.

Trekking Poles: Most trekking poles are used as a pair, one in each hand, however, it's possible to use one trekking pole by itself. These poles look more athletic than other mobility aids, which is why they're a first choice when someone is dabbling with mobility aids. They can be a great way to get walking support and maintain balance without the stigma of using a typical mobility aid.

Cane: This provides slightly more support than a trekking pole since the cane tip is broader. A cane is often used on one side of the body, making this a common mobility aid for those requiring minimal support. Since it isn't cumbersome, a cane is another great option if you're brand new to mobility aids. Some people use two canes (one in each hand) for more support. If two canes is your thing, consider the Lofstrand forearm crutches. One of my favorite brands for canes is NeoWalk Walking Sticks.

Most people aren't aware of the proper way to use a single trekking pole or cane, which is to hold it on the opposite side of the weaker leg. For example, if your left leg is weaker than your right, hold the cane in your right hand. Then, as you're walking, make sure your right hand is placing the cane on your walking surface (floor, pavement, etc.) at the same time your body weight is on your left leg. This allows you to transfer body weight from the weaker leg to the stronger side by putting the weight through the cane or trekking pole. If you held the cane on the same side as your weak leg, then all of your body weight would go to the weaker side of your body, potentially causing a fall or pain. This concept doesn't apply to a walker or rollator since your hands hold onto stationary handles.

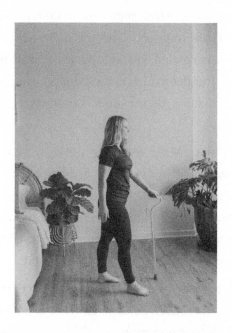

With that said, if you've been using a cane or a trekking pole for many years in the "wrong" hand and using it in the "correct" hand feels unstable, use it in the way that makes you feel safest. Similarly, if you have hand weakness, tightness, or pain preventing you from using the aid on the "correct" side, please use the aid on the opposite side. A mobility aid should make you feel more stable, safe and in control, so make adjustments if my recommendations don't fit your needs.

Rollator: Rollators offer more support than a cane or trekking pole, and the wheels allow for smooth travel without breaking your stride. Don't worry, they do come with brakes. There are three-wheeled and four-wheeled rollators. Generally, three-wheeled rollators come with a basket and four-wheeled rollators have a seat with or without a basket. Four-wheeled rollators are great for walking long distances where you may want to take a rest on the seat. Most rollators are collapsible and can easily be transported to and from the car and house. If you're commuting, get a rollator light enough to maneuver it. byACRE offers sturdy, lightweight rollators.

Wheelchair: This is often used when the body needs more rest. It can be used as your primary form of mobility or just on days when you don't have enough energy, strength, or balance to support your walking. Or, save your energy by using a wheelchair in an airport as you travel through the terminal and to the gate. This conserves your energy to move about once you reach your destination. There are several types of wheelchairs, including manual chairs (where you control the chair by pushing the wheels) or power chairs (which are controlled via a joystick) or transport chairs (which are designed to be pushed by someone else).

Emily, a MSing Link member, uses a mix of three mobility aids depending on how her body is feeling each day: a manual wheelchair, rollator, and one or two trekking poles. She chooses which aid to use based on her energy level, strength and stamina, and endurance. Some days, Emily uses a single trekking pole and other times she uses her rollator. Her wheelchair is used for the days or moments when walking requires more energy and strength than she has to give. Emily has used her wheelchair, rollator, and cane all in one day.

There are no rules. Using a wheelchair doesn't mean you can't walk. Why not empower yourself with a toolbox of mobility aids to make life easier?

How to Measure a Mobility Aid to Your Body

If you're using trekking poles, there are two options for height adjustments. The first option is to bend your elbows, placed against the side of your body, at 90 degrees. The handles of the trekking pole should be about one fist length above your hand. The second option is to arrange the trekking pole handles about halfway between your waist and your hips. For a video demonstrating how to adjust and use trekking poles, head over to my YouTube page.

If you're using a cane, walker, or rollator, stand up tall with your arms down by your side. The handle of the aid should be at the height of your wrist bone. This height allows you to use the mobility aid most effectively. If you've been using your aid at a different height for many years and my suggestion is uncomfortable or makes you unsteady, then please use a height that's safe and comfortable for you.

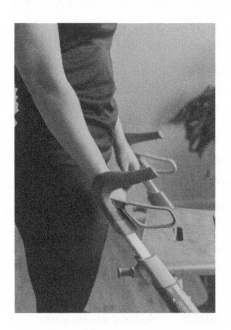
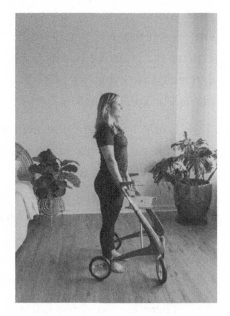

How to Not Become Dependent on a Mobility Aid

If you're worried that using a mobility aid will mean that you won't be able to walk without one, here's a tip for you. Put less than 50 percent of your body weight through the aid while standing or walking. This will lessen the likelihood of slipping or falling and train your brain to understand that the aid is there for support and guidance. Your brain won't view it as a necessity. The more weight you put through your arms on your aid, the more your brain will rewire itself to think you *need* it, resulting in dependency on the aid. You'll also have less shoulder, elbow, or wrist pain from putting less weight through your upper body.

Ankle Foot Orthosis (AFO) and Electrical Stimulation

Ankle Foot Orthosis (AFO) is an ankle brace worn in your shoe that aims to reduce drop foot by limiting the amount of movement in your ankle. They can be made out of various materials but the most common are carbon fiber and plastic. Many factors are considered when determining which AFO design is best for you and your goals. Some AFOs are better for people without strength or movement in their ankles while others are better for people with some strength and mobility in their ankles. Some AFOs are best for people who are looking to run, and others are better for people who will only be using them to walk. Go to an orthotist to test several types and find the best one for your needs. Orthotists are specialists who help navigate various types of AFOs, evaluate walking with and without the AFOs, and ultimately assist in choosing the best one for you.

If you're an AFO user, wear the AFO as often as needed to remain safe, but not more than that. This is done to avoid additional weakness, since you aren't using your ankle muscles as much as you do without the AFO. So, if your drop foot isn't affecting you one day, don't wear the AFO. Or if you need the AFO in the afternoon or later in the day since your muscles are fatigued at that time, use the AFO during those time periods, but not all day. We want your ankle to remain strong while using the AFO for safety.

When it comes to exercising with an AFO, there are two options: on or off. If you're someone who uses an AFO and you feel very unsteady or weak without the AFO on, then you should exercise with the AFO on. However, if you're able to move around safely without the AFO on, my preference is that you don't wear the AFO while exercising. This allows full use of your neural pathways and ankle muscles to improve ankle strength and balance.

> "If you're able to move around safely without an Ankle Foot Orthosis (AFO), don't wear it while exercising. This allows full use of your neural pathways and ankle muscles to improve ankle strength and balance."

Dawn, a MSing Link member, had used an AFO for one year. Her foot drop had improved while wearing the brace, but then she started swinging/circumducting her hip more often. The reason? Her leg muscles weakened due to relying on the AFO. Her weakness led to impairments in other body parts, like her hip and knee. Once she started performing MSing Link strengthening exercises without the AFO, she regained knee and hip balance. And she didn't need the AFO as often. Now, Dawn only uses the AFO on days when she needs more assistance.

Some of my favorite AFO alternates are ankle braces, including the Dictus Band, Elevate 360 Drop Foot Brace, Saebo Foot Drop band, and Foot Up Brace. A strap attaches around your ankle and a rubber band or string that extends to clips in the eyelets of your shoe. The rubber band and string assist in lifting your ankle when walking. The biggest difference between an AFO and these braces is that an AFO works by preventing the undesired movement of your ankle falling downward; and the ankle braces assist with the desired movement of lifting your ankle.

Another alternative aid is electrical stimulation devices like the Walk Aide, Bioness, Neubie, PONS, or Cionic Neural Sleeve. All of these devices use a current (either direct, alternate, or pulsed) to activate neural pathways and muscles. These are ideal for people looking to improve drop foot, since the muscles these devices stimulate assist with lifting the ankle and bending the knee.

Some electrical stimulation devices can be used while walking throughout the day while others are intended for exercise only. Similar to AFOs, I suggest exercising without the electrical stimulation device, so you can focus on strengthening neural pathways and muscles without assistance. However, it's a good idea to exercise with the device, too. Aim for 50 percent of exercise without assistance from the stimulation device and 50 percent with assistance. If you only exercise while wearing the device, you may never be able to activate your muscles without assistance, resulting in dependency on the device.

Siobhan, a MSing Link member, had been using Bioness, an electrical stimulation device, for several years. At first, it greatly improved her drop foot, but after a while, when she walked around the house or outdoors without the device, her walking got worse. One likely reason is that she'd trained her muscles to work only when they had assistance from the stimulation. To combat this, she performed the MSing Link hip, knee, and ankle strengthening exercises without the device, and after several months, she was able to walk without the Bioness.

KEY TAKEAWAYS

1 Mobility aids are designed to help you stay independent and mobile.

2 It's okay to use different or multiple varieties of mobility aids, based on how you're feeling day- to-day.

3 Ankle Foot Orthosis (AFO), ankle braces, and electrical stimulation are tools used to reduce drop foot. These can be used in addition to a mobility aid or on their own.

4 Have hope! There are so many tools out there to assist you!

RESOURCES

• The MSing Link podcast episode No. 11, "Mobility Aids - The Best Options for You!"

• For more of my favorite tools, including the ones mentioned here, go to my Amazon affiliate account: https://www.amazon.com/shop/doctor.gretchen

CHAPTER 10

Your Biggest Enemy
Is Yourself

Here's a little secret: Making long-lasting changes and improvements require the appropriate treatment and exercise as well as consistency and the right mindset. The majority of my clients share what their inner critic says to them while they're exercising. It's often things like, "Really, Stacy ... that's *all* you can do? You're hardly exercising. This isn't worth it and it won't make a difference." In Rachel's case, her inner critic kept saying, "You used to do *so* much more than what you're doing now. It's pathetic that this little movement is all you can do."

Unfortunately, these unkind thoughts are completely normal, but you can't let them win. These thoughts will lead to feeling discouraged, disappointed, and defeated. And guess what action you take when you're feeling that way? No action. No exercise. No results.

I want you to picture yourself sitting at your kitchen table with a bright yellow lemon sitting on a cutting board right in front of you. The lemon looks plump and juicy and as you pick it up, you smell a strong citrus scent and can feel that it's firm and ready to use. You put the lemon back on the cutting board and pick up a knife. Slowly, you cut the lemon and as soon as the knife pierces the lemon rind, you see lemon juice squirt out of the lemon. As you continue to cut, you see a pool of lemon juice on the cutting board along with some of the seeds. The strong citrus aroma intensifies as it stings your nostrils. Once the lemon is cut, you cut it again into quarters, making even more juice pool on the cutting board. Then, you pick up one piece and bite into it. Your jaw tightens as the sourness kicks into high gear and your taste buds perk up, your lips pucker, and your nose squints.

Did you start to salivate at any point while envisioning cutting or biting into the lemon? Did you make any faces to show disgust for biting the lemon? Psychiatrist Florence Hagenmuller of University of Zurich and others' research in 2014 found that most people would have had one or both of the previous reactions after reading that story, which proves our mindset plays a role in our physical body. A bodily function, like salivation, occurred simply from thinking about biting into a lemon. Applying this same theory to exercising, your thoughts can result in physical action or inaction. If your mindset believes you can't get stronger, you probably won't get stronger. A negative mindset might cause someone to be inconsistent with their exercise routine or avoid it altogether because they don't believe it will make a difference. And as we all know, if you're not consistent, you won't see any changes. If your mindset says you can improve your strength, you probably will, since you'll also stay more consistent and motivated. Now, of course, there are some important considerations as MS can have a mind of its own and no matter how hard you work, there is a possibility it may not make a difference due to disease progression. But there's also a good chance it will make a difference, even with disease progression. My clients with MS realize the possibilities and see real change when they have hope, believe, and stay consistent.

How to Get on Track and Stay Consistent for the Long Haul

Create a powerful "why" statement. When movement becomes challenging and your life is busy, it's easy to let exercise slip off the daily to-do list, which is why having a powerful reason to exercise is so important. Without a why, exercise can feel like an option rather than a non-negotiable priority. The goal is to create a reason so powerful it makes you feel emotional. At first glance, your reason behind exercising consistently may be to get stronger or to walk better. While those are great goals, they often aren't motivating enough to get you moving on the hard days, which, let's be honest, may be most days. The best way to create a why statement is to ask yourself "why do I want to exercise consistently?" Once you answer, ask yourself "why?" again. Repeat this process until you have an answer that moves you emotionally and physically.

MSing Link member Lydia thought she knew which exercises were aligned with her goals, but she wasn't motivated to do them. I took Lydia through the exercise of creating a strong why. Here's how it went:

Me: "Why is exercise important to you?"

Lydia: "I want to get stronger."

Me: "Why do you want to get stronger?"

Lydia: "So I can maintain my independence."

Me: "Why do you want to maintain your independence?"

Lydia: "So I can take care of myself and my son."

Me: "Why do you want to be able to take care of yourself and your son?"

Lydia: "So my son can have fun experiences with me, like trick or treating."

Me: "Why do you want to have fun experiences with your son?"

Lydia: "So I can be a part of his life."

BAM! How powerful is that? Lydia's why statement went from being "I want to exercise to be stronger" to "I want to exercise so that I can be part of my son's life." Which one do you think will motivate her to get out of bed in the morning and prioritize her exercise? The latter, of course.

Lydia and I also discussed other major life events, like walking down the aisle at her son's wedding, which was years away. After this conversation, Lydia learned to associate exercise with being part of her son's life. When I checked in a few months later, she had stayed consistent with her exercise plan every week.

MSing Link member, Heather, used to be a marathoner, and a rock climber and loved staying active. Her MS symptoms hit quickly and she noticed a rapid decline in her ability to walk and get outside of her house. We developed an exercise program that included several seated and a few standing exercises. Heather said when she was exercising, she heard her inner voice saying, "This is NOTHING compared to what I used to do ... this is pointless." She tried to kick that inner voice to the curb, but it kept coming back to discourage her. I told her to envision herself hugging that inner voice instead of giving it the boot. Then, I shared what she might tell that inner voice, which was: It's okay to feel discouraged, hurt and hopeless - I understand. Once Heather did that, it was time to change the narrative and remind herself that those exercises are a step toward her goals, no matter if they felt far away. Heather utilized this practice daily and she became more consistent (over time) developing a better relationship with exercise that left her feeling motivated and hopeful.

Pick one thing and start small. If you aren't exercising consistently or feel lost, getting started can be daunting. The best way to get started is to start small. While you may have set a goal of exercising five days per week for 30 minutes per day, if that schedule is new to you, it might be hard to stick to, especially considering any fatigue that comes along with introducing new movement patterns. Pick one exercise and do it for 10 repetitions one day this week. That's it. Once you're done, you don't have to exercise again until next week. Once you do this for several weeks, you'll feel able to do a second set of 10 repetitions of the exercise. Or maybe you'd like to add a second exercise. Or do the exercise two days a week instead of one day. Most progress comes from starting at a point that feels very attainable. So while it may feel useless to do just one exercise one day per week, it will start to add up over time. Getting started is the first step to seeing long-term progress. Start small and add more movements when you can.

Pick a schedule that makes sense for you. Dr. Bernard Duvivier from Maastricht University Medical Center and numerous other researchers have proven that exercising throughout the day is as effective as exercising all at once. Don't pressure yourself to exercise for 40 minutes in one sitting, if that doesn't work for your energy levels or your busy schedule. Trust that exercising for five minutes many times throughout the day will add up to your cumulative exercise time for the day, and you will see results, even if you don't break a sweat. And if you truly don't have time to exercise one day, don't forget daily movement counts as exercise, too. Unloading the dishwasher, grabbing the mail, walking around the house, getting dressed, showering, and walking to and from work counts too.

Think positive thoughts before, during, and after. If you're focusing on negative fear-based thoughts while exercising, you will *not* enjoy it. It'll make you feel defeated, hopeless, and less than. Those thoughts will almost always lead to falling off the wagon and constantly restarting your exercise routine. How often do we stick to routines that don't make us feel good? Rarely. So change the narrative! Focus on your why, the good things exercise can bring, the goals you'll reach, and the firm belief that what you're doing *is* enough to see improvement. These positive thoughts are more likely to form a positive association with exercise. You'll stay consistent with something that makes you feel hopeful and reminds you of your goals.

Don't forget your proof. You have plenty of life examples of staying consistent even though it was challenging or you didn't believe you could do it. This is proof that you can reach other goals, like staying consistent with exercise and daily movement, too. Make a list of your proof and pull it out anytime doubt creeps up. Remember, everything counts!

Here are some activities and tasks that require consistency:

- passing exams
- getting a degree
- learning a new language
- knocking out the driver's test
- quitting smoking
- traveling
- having long-lasting relationships
- completing a project
- taking your medication
- staying hydrated

Surround yourself with positive success stories and personal development. If you're surrounded by people who make you feel like you can't improve, it will be a lot harder to get started and stay on track. Read and/or listen to success stories, such as the ones in this book; locate research that supports the possibility of neuroplasticity; get an accountability partner; and find support online. The MSing

Link is a great opportunity to get all of these in one place. It includes support from our accountability group, research from MS experts, and tons of MS-specific exercises based on neuroplasticity.

The Compound Effect

Are you familiar with the Aesop Fable, "The Frog in The Milk Pail"? If not, allow me to introduce it to you. A frog hopped around a farmyard looking for good things to eat and found wonderfully juicy insects, flies, mosquitos, and spiders. As he approached each one, he gulped it down. As the frog hopped around finding these insects, he explored new territory and witnessed a cricket hop into a milk shed, through a door, up onto a milk stool, over to a tabletop, up onto a window ledge, and out the window.

The frog was intrigued, so he followed the cricket, but instead of making it out the window, he fell into the milk pail, which was filled halfway with fresh milk. The milk level was too low and the sides of the pail were too high for him to climb out, he was stuck. The frog tired from kicking and swimming in circles, so he stopped to rest but in doing so, he sank to the bottom of the pail. He used his legs to push off the bottom of the pail and swam his way up to the surface. He was afraid of sinking again, but he was also so tired. All he wanted was to rest, but every time he quit kicking, he started to drown.

But the frog made a decision to not give into his fear or his tired legs. He took a big breath and began kicking endlessly until the milk began to turn thicker. At first, this made the kicking and swimming harder than ever, but he did not give up. Eventually, the milk turned thick enough that the frog could stand up on top of it, the milk had turned into butter from the frog's kicking and swimming! The frog was then able to climb out to safety.

I think we can apply this challenge-turned-victory into our daily life. When things get tough and we've had enough, take a big breath and keep moving forward in any way you can. For the frog, each kick seemed meaningless, but over time it compounded. This applies to all areas of our life including exercise, learning, finances, etc. This concept allows neuroplasticity to improve our walking, strength & balance!

To get started with the compound effect, choose a small task, something you can commit to daily, for example exercising for ten minutes. The rest is simple, perform a small task every day. Over the course of time, you'll see real results, one step at a time.

KEY TAKEAWAYS

1. Our mindset has a direct effect on our physical bodies.

2. Observe your thoughts around exercise. If they're negative, change them to inspirational thoughts. Create a meaningful reason (your "why") to exercise and remind yourself of it often.

3. Pick one or two strategies of the six listed in this chapter to get on track and stay consistent; start implementing them today.

4. Every positive action for your body will compound over time. Trust the process.

5. Have hope! Believe in yourself. You can do this.

RESOURCES

The MSing Link podcast episodes:

- Episode No. 31, "Goal Setting and Staying Consistent"
- Episode No 72, "What Does Consistency Really Mean?"
- Episode No. 36, "Compound Effect"
- Episode No. 54, "Your Inner Self Critic"

TOP FAQs

You've just learned many exercises and strategies to improve your strength, walking, balance, and day-to-day mobility. However, if you're thinking, "Yeah, but ... I can't do that," or "Yes, but that's not how my body moves," this section troubleshoots some of the most common movements or situations preventing people with MS from living life to the fullest.

1. **Q: I can't exercise for 30 minutes. Is it still worth it to exercise for less than 30 minutes?**

   A: As you now know, MS research shows that exercising throughout the day is just as effective as exercising all at once. If you can exercise for 5 minutes at a time, attempt to do that 6 times throughout the day, totaling 30 cumulative minutes of exercise. Or, exercise for 3 minutes, 5 times per day. Something is better than nothing. The majority of MSing Link members exercise throughout the day at their desk, kitchen table, and the sofa! Using this strategy, they see amazing results such as walking longer distances, less tripping and falling, more ease with climbing stairs, and less difficulty getting into and out of the car. Daily movements, like getting dressed, showering, and cooking count as exercise! Some exercise and movement is better than none.

2. Q: I plop down/fall backward when I sit down or attempt to stand up.

A: Most times, this isn't connected to your strength (or lack thereof), but shoulder and hip alignment! If your waist and shoulders are upright, you're more likely to fall backward. The best strategy to stay stable when sitting down or standing up is to keep your hips hinged and your shoulders forward until you're in the desired position. When sitting down, take your buttock backward and bring your shoulders forward, then bend your knees until your bottom touches the chair. Once you're sitting, lift your shoulders so you're sitting upright. If you bring your shoulders back too quickly, you'll plop down. Similarly, when you stand up, keep your shoulders forward and buttock back until your knees are straight, THEN bring your hips forward and stand upright.

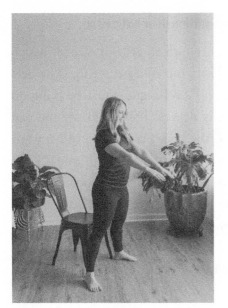

Step 1 - Stand with wide stance

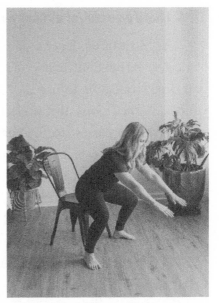

Step 2 - Hinge Forward; keep your shoulders forward as you bend your knees until you're sitting on the chair.

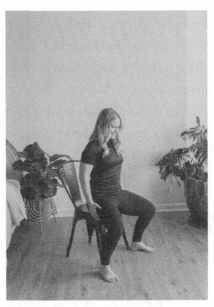

Step 3 - Once your bottom is touching the chair, sit up tall.

3. Q: I have pain and/or difficulty when getting in or out of bed.

A: Most of us depend on core strength to get out of bed, which can cause extreme difficulty and/or back, hip, and neck pain. The best pain-free strategy is to use the "log roll" technique. Start by lying on your back then cross the ankle that is nearest the middle of the bed over the ankle closest to the edge of the bed. From here, roll toward the outside of the bed, using your elbows to help push you in the appropriate direction. Once you're lying on your side, scoot your feet off the bed, place both hands on the bed and push yourself upright at the same time that your feet and lower legs descend toward the floor. You can use this same technique in reverse for getting into bed pain-free. This technique can also be used if you have difficulty getting on or off the couch or MRI table.

4. Q: I touch walls or furniture when I walk. Is this okay?

A: In the physical therapy world, this is called "wall walking" or "furniture walking." This is not a good habit since it can lead to falling, especially if you reach for a wall or furniture outside of your home. My favorite way to reduce wall and furniture walking is to practice walking while standing close to a wall, but not touching the wall. Once you feel safe, practice walking slightly further away from the wall. Keep repeating this until you're able to practice walking in the middle of a room. This may take several weeks or several months to work up to and can be performed with or without a mobility aid.

5. Q: One of my legs is weaker than the other, should I strengthen my weak side instead of both sides?

A: Any exercise you perform on your stronger side will keep those neural pathways strong, which is what we want! I always suggest exercising equally on your weak side and strong side. This will strengthen your muscles and your neural pathways. The stronger your neural pathways are, the less likely you'll feel weakness and limitations from a relapse or progression.

6.   Q: I can't walk on uneven ground, what should I do?

A: Walking on uneven ground requires three things: strength, balance, and mindset/confidence. One of the best exercises is to walk on uneven ground using exaggerated steps with a mobility aid. This will allow you to improve your strength and balance on uneven surfaces in addition to training your mind that this activity is possible for you. If you never practice walking on uneven ground, your mind will likely panic when you are in a position that requires you to walk on grass, cobblestone, pebbles, sand, sidewalk, etc. When your mind panics, your body follows suit and doesn't cooperate, often resulting in tightening muscles, weakness, or falling. Practicing walking on these surfaces trains your mind to believe you're capable of doing it. If you believe you can do it, your body is more likely to accomplish the task.

7.   Q: I use my arms to lift my leg into a car, bed, bathtub, etc. How do I fix this?

A: Using your arms to lift your leg often occurs for two reasons—weak hip flexors and habit. Practice the seated marching exercise as often as possible with good quality. Bonus points if you practice it in the exact location you need to use it, such as in your car, at the edge of your bed, or the edge of the bathtub. Also, you've probably been using your arms to lift your legs for several years, meaning this is a strong habit that must be broken. Anytime you're in a position where you normally use your arms to lift your leg, choose to attempt to lift using your leg strength instead.

The most common follow-up statement when I share the answer above is: "But ... my leg doesn't lift when I attempt to lift it."

That's okay. It takes time to build strength, which is what you're doing by practicing the marching exercise. This trains your brain to get rid of the old habit and create a new one, even if your leg doesn't lift. I like to implement my "rule of two," which means you should attempt to lift your leg without your arms twice. If it doesn't lift by the second time, go ahead and use your arms to assist. This way, you're retraining your brain to attempt to use your leg muscles instead of your arms, but you're also not slowing yourself down to the point where you can't go about your day-to-day life.

The rule of two applies any time you're working on creating new habits that may slow you down. For example, if you have a goal of bending your knee more when you're walking, but you're in a rush and need to go to the bathroom, attempt to bend your knee twice. If it doesn't work, go ahead and get to the bathroom in whatever way you can.

8.   Q: I struggle to stand up from the floor. How can I do this safely?

A: I have two favorite ways to stand up from the floor safely. If possible, scoot close to sturdy furniture that you can use to help you stand up if needed.

Option No. 1: The Lunge: Start sitting upright with your legs out in front of you. Roll toward your stronger side until you're on your hands and knees. If possible, place one or both hands on a couch or nearby furniture so that you can assume a tall-kneeling position. Pick up your stronger leg and place it in front of you (this may take several steps, instead of one big swoop). You should now have one foot on the floor and the opposite knee on the floor. From here, straighten both knees while pushing up through your hands on the couch/chair/ furniture. Once you're standing, put more body weight through the front leg and move your back leg forward until you're standing upright. Ideally, do this next to a piece of furniture, so you can use your arms to assist.

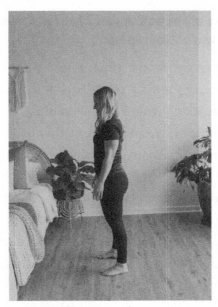

7 - **Stand up tall**

Disclaimer: Whichever option you choose, this is challenging and takes practice. Pick an option that feels more doable for you and practice it as an exercise so you can get stronger with this movement.

9. Q: I can't strengthen my legs because my balance is so bad. What should I do?

A: Mobility aids can be your best friend for exercising. If poor balance is a problem, hold onto a trekking pole, cane, walker or rollator. This allows you to focus on strengthening your muscles without worrying about balance. Hold on as lightly as possible, instead of holding on for dear life. Remember, strength and balance training are two different types of exercise. You should focus on strength and balance separately, not at the same time, so neither is compromised.

10. Q: My back hurts when I walk and/or when I pick something up off the floor or when I twist. What can I do?

A: Ninety percent of the time when someone has MS-related back pain, it's caused by a weak core. Two simple tricks to reduce this type of back pain is to tighten the abdominal and gluteal muscles. Utilize the core exercises you learned in this book. When tightening your abdominal muscles, focus on using your belly muscles to pull your belly button back toward your spine. This is different than just sucking in. When tightening your gluteal muscles, focus on squeezing a quarter between your buttock. Activating these two muscle groups will help stabilize you and reduce the likelihood of other muscles being overworked, which causes pain. If your back pain is due to an injury, see a physical therapist and/or primary care doctor.

You did it!

You now have all the exercises and tools to help you feel more confident in your exercise routine and see real improvements in your day-to-day mobility!

So ... what's next for you? Keep up your momentum and start implementing these exercises and strategies in my free 5 Day MS Strength Challenge! In this challenge you'll get a review of some of the most important concepts you learned in this book, like neuroplasticity, functional exercises to improve walking, how to fit exercising into your day, and how to stay consistent. Plus, you'll have one challenge each day to help you take action towards the goals you're working towards.

You don't have to do this alone. I'm here to help! To access my free 5 Day MS Strength challenge, go here:

https://www.doctorgretchenhawley.com/MSChallenge

Resources

The resources below will teach you the best exercises and strategies to meet your goals:

1. **Access a pdf and video demonstration of all of the exercises in this book:** https://www.doctorgretchenhawley.com/bookpdf

2. **The MSing Link Podcast:**

   Check in with Dr. Gretchen weekly as she chats about the newest therapies, research, exercises, and symptom management strategies. You'll also hear from outstanding guests, including MS neurologists, dieticians, sleep experts, neuro scientists, and more.

   https://www.doctorgretchenhawley.com/podcasts/the-msing-link

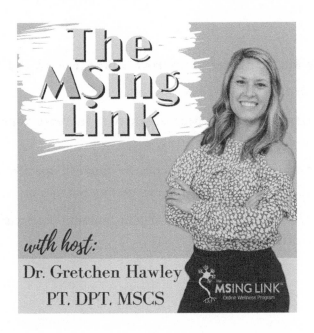

3. The MSing Link App (iOS & Android):

This is your one-stop shop to track your exercises and symptoms, watch MS-specific exercise videos, access Dr. Gretchen's YouTube videos and podcast, and chat with the community.

The MSing Link App (iOS): https://apps.apple.com/us/app/the-msing-link/id1606973076

The MSing Link App (Android): https://play.google.com/store/apps/details?id=com.x25e14b93419.app&hl=en_US&gl=US

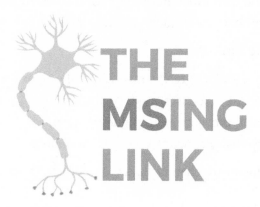

4. 5-Day MS Challenge to Improve Your Strength and Walking:

In this free 5 day challenge, you'll learn:

- How you can use neuroplasticity to **increase your strength and improve mobility**!

- Various functional exercises to **improve specific activities** (i.e. walking, stair climbing, getting out of a car, etc.).

- The amount of time you should commit to **exercising to see a difference**.

- How to **fit MS-specific exercises into your day**.

- How to **stay consistent** with your exercise routine.

https://www.doctorgretchenhawley.com/MSChallenge

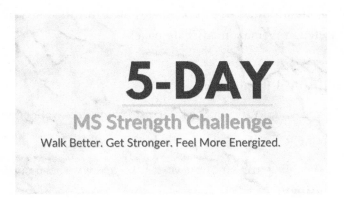

5. MS-Specific Walking Webinar:

In this one-hour webinar, Dr. Gretchen will educate you on MS-specific physical therapy compared to "traditional" physical therapy. You'll see her demonstrate every component of walking, including tons of exercises to implement into your daily routine right away!

https://www.doctorgretchenhawley.com/walking-webinar

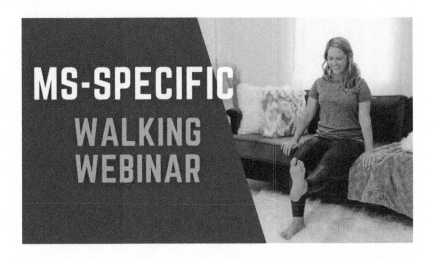

6. **Products & Helpful Tools:** https://www.amazon.com/shop/doctor. gretchen

Find all of the products and tools mentioned in this book, plus more, on Dr. Gretchen's Amazon Affiliate page!

7. **Mobility Aid Resources:**

- NeoWalk Walking Stick: https://www.neo-walk.com/

- byACRE rollator: https://www.byacre.com/

- Thermapparel Cooling Vest: https://www.thermapparel.com/ msinglink

WORK WITH
DR. GRETCHEN HAWLEY
PT, DPT, MSCS

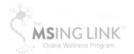

The MSing Link Online MS Wellness Program:

If you want to work directly with Dr. Gretchen, this membership is for you! The MSing Link Online MS Wellness Program is for people with MS who want to feel seen, heard, and supported while feeling confident in their exercise routine. You'll get access to 150+ MS-specific exercises and classes, daily guides and programs sharing which exercises to do each day, and plenty of opportunities to get your questions answered from Dr. Gretchen and other MS experts. This wellness program will help you reach your goals of improved walking quality and stamina, stair climbing, less tripping, and more confidence in your mobility. Learn more at the link below:

https://www.doctorgretchenhawley.com/TheMSingLink

Work 1:1 with Dr. Gretchen Hawley PT, DPT, MSCS

Looking for personalized coaching through your goals? Apply to work 1:1 with me here:

https://www.doctorgretchenhawley.com/assessments/2147688291

Thank you so much for reading my book! If this book has added value to your life, if you feel like you're more empowered after reading it, and if you see that *The MSing Link's* exercises and strategies can be a new beginning for you to take your exercise routine and symptom management to the next level, please consider paying it forward by leaving a review here:

https://www.doctorgretchenhawley.com/bookreview

It would mean the world to me to have *The MSing Link* spread far and wide to help as many people with MS as possible take back control and feel more hope towards their journey with MS.

Acknowledgments

Having an idea and turning it into a book is as hard as it sounds. The experience was both challenging and rewarding. I want to thank the individuals who helped make this happen.

I'm eternally grateful for my parents, Ted and Patricia, who taught me discipline and that anything is achievable with hard work. You encouraged me to chase my dreams, even if that meant moving seven-plus hours away for 10 years. I'll never forget your unshakable belief in me when I announced my plan to start my own company to fulfill a need in the MS community. You believed in me from day one and it's the reason I'm successful today. A special thank you to my mom who was my first beta reader and for sharing your feedback and copy edits. Thank you from the bottom of my heart.

I'd like to thank my husband, Jeff, for always being my biggest cheerleader. From watching every single YouTube video, liking every Instagram post, listening to all of my podcast episodes, you always encourage my drive to help others. Your support makes me feel like my book, online programs, and social media content is changing the world. I love doing life with you.

A huge thank you to my twin sister, Samantha, who has been a huge part of The MSing Link and every business decision. You were sitting by my side at a bar in Nashville as we brainstormed what would eventually become The MSing Link. You have been an integral part of every program, course, and content production I've developed, including this book. Our business meetings, dance breaks, and strategy sessions mean the world to me. Thank you for everything.

Thank you to my older sister, Gillian, for showing me what going after your dreams look like. Your determination and drive are unmatched. You've led by example, giving me the courage to dream bigger and not be afraid to change the course when I've outgrown the old one. Thank you for being a great role model.

I'd like to thank my MSing Link members for trusting and believing in me as your guide and for your consistent effort in working on yourself and your goals. Your testimonials give hope to so many and are a true testament that hard work pays off. Your feedback on my exercises and strategies (which you've never learned before!) gave me the drive to write this book. Your words are fuel as I help as many people with MS who aren't receiving the knowledge they need to feel more confident and reach their goals. I appreciate all of our conversations and the community we've built together.

I'd like to thank my social media followers for helping me create this book! Thank you for your constant feedback about topics, activities, pictures and the book cover. This book was designed for people with MS, so your commentary was invaluable!

A big shout out to my first mentor and colleague, Courtney Capwell PT, DPT, MSCS. From helping me study for the MS Certification exam, to showing me the ropes with MS physical therapy treatments, your guidance has been key in the way I educate and treat my clients. You showed me what being a passionate healthcare professional and advocate looks like and it's made a lasting impression. I aim to bring that same passion to my work.

I'm forever grateful to Taiia Smart Young, my book coach, Kelsea Koenreich, my business coach, and my publishing team for your editorial help, keen insight, and ongoing support in bringing my words to life. Your guidance in creating this book was crucial and I've learned so much!

Last but not least, a shout-out to my dogs, Finn and Stanley, for cuddling next to me as I wrote this book. My love language is physical touch, so your cuddles helped me feel loved, calm and centered as I wrote this book. I hope every reader feels this, too.

About the Author

D r. Gretchen is a physical therapist and Multiple Sclerosis Certified Specialist. She is the founder and creator of The MSing Link, an online program offering global services to help people with MS feel more confident in their strength, walking, and daily activities. Her groundbreaking exercises and strategies utilize neuroplasticity, targeting improvements in the neural pathways in the brain and spinal cord as well as muscles. Dr. Gretchen has been featured in *Forbes*, *National MS Society*, *Overcoming MS*, *MS-UK*, and *MS Views and News*. Dr. Gretchen has frequently appeared on TV including 13 WHAM, WGRZ, and WIVB. She is a frequent presenter at national and international MS conferences.

You can find Dr. Gretchen in the following places:

Dr. Gretchen's Services: https://www.doctorgretchenhawley.com

The MSing Link: https://www.doctorgretchenhawley.com/ TheMSingLink

YouTube: https://www.youtube.com/c/DoctorGretchenHawley

Instagram: https://www.instagram.com/doctor.gretchen

TikTok: https://www.tiktok.com/@drgretchenpt

Facebook: https://www.facebook.com/groups/MSWellness

The MSing Link podcast: https://www.doctorgretchenhawley.com/ podcasts/the-msing-link

The MSing Link app (Android): https://play.google.com/store/apps/ details?id=com.x25e14b93419.app&hl=en_US&gl=US

The MSing Link app (iOS): https://apps.apple.com/us/app/the-msing-link/id1606973076

Made in United States
North Haven, CT
30 October 2023

43363016R00104